Beyond the smile

Photographs may be used as an adjunct to many kinds of therapy; in her own practice Linda Berman found that patients often brought photographs of their own accord. This encouraged her to think about what lay behind the photographs in the family album, and how they could best be used to help her patients. *Beyond the Smile* is the record of her personal journey, an exploration of the meanings of photographs and an examination of the ways in which photographs can enhance the effectiveness of a psychotherapy session.

The book focuses on the relationship between the photograph and the self and stresses the need for the therapist to understand his or her own personal images before approaching those of others. Individual case studies, with appropriate illustrations, show how photographs can highlight the themes within the patient's internal and external worlds, stimulating new awareness of interactional patterns and illuminating in a very personal way how the past influences the present. Linda Berman shows how photographs can be incorporated successfully into many therapeutic styles and settings and demonstrates how therapists may use their own personal photographs to further self-development.

Beyond the Smile will be of great value to students and professionals in pyschotherapy, psychology and counselling, and to all those interested in the hidden messages behind the photographic image.

Linda Berman is a psychotherapist and marital therapist in private practice.

Beyond the smile: the therapeutic use of the photograph

Linda Berman

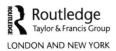 Routledge
Taylor & Francis Group

LONDON AND NEW YORK

For Paul, Richard and Steven

First published in 1993
by Routledge
27 Church Road, Hove East Sussex BN3 2FA
711 Third Avenue, New York, NY 10017

Routledge is an imprint of the Taylor & Francis Group, an informa business

© 1993 Linda Berman

Typeset in Times by J&L Composition Ltd, Filey, North Yorkshire

British Library Cataloguing in Publication Data
A catalogue record for this book is available from the British Library

ISBN 0–415–06763–4

Contents

Preface   vi
Acknowledgements   ix

1 Photographs in everyday life   1

2 'I am here, I am there': paradoxes, contradictions and ambiguities
  within the photograph   23

3 Using photographs in therapy: some general principles   51

4 A clinical example: Jane   82

5 A closer look at the family album: searching for clues to the past 105

6 The search continues: exploring images of interaction   122

7 Who can benefit?   146

8 'Can it really be me?' Photographs and the self   174

  Conclusion   203
  Notes   204
  Bibliography   206
  Further reading   209
  Name index   210
  Subject index   212

Preface

During my work as a therapist, many patients have brought to me photographs of parents, spouses, siblings, children. Often, having responded with interest, I felt uncertain about using them therapeutically and would be left with a sense of missed opportunity. Gradually, however, I began to explore ways in which the photographs could be utilised in the session and my interest in them began to grow and 'develop' within my own clinical practice.

My research widened out considerably as I contemplated writing this book, leading me into new and exciting areas. Each new discovery, each step, led me further into the fascinating and complex and uncertain world of photographs as therapy.

I feel privileged to have been allowed into several people's personal worlds through sharing their photographs. I have 'met' their relatives and friends and 'watched' them through the growing up process. I have shared the intense pain and joy as repressed memories cascade through time into consciousness, and I have witnessed the subsequent dawning of new insight.

My desire to produce this book was born out of a wish to communicate how intrinsically *useful* photographs are, not only in therapy, but also in our lives generally. My material comes from both inside and outside the psychotherapy situation, reflecting the fact that photographs are also meaningful in our everyday lives. It is, however, important to diffentiate at the outset between the use of photographs in our lives generally, perhaps for purposes of memory and nostalgia, and their use in therapy. Whilst the former may provide us with a therapeutic experience, it is not therapy; photographic exploration within the accepting yet analytical atmosphere of the therapy session is a very different experience. The patient is frequently surprised when photographs that have been perused many times at home suddenly take on a whole new meaning in therapy.

While the main focus of the book is on the use of photographs in psychoanalytic psychotherapy, I hope that it will also be of interest to therapists of all disciplines and approaches and to anyone who is curious about how to look at photographs with an eye to their psychological meaning.

Much has been written about photographs, but there is relatively little about their use in therapy, especially in Britain. There are certainly therapists of all kinds using photographs to help their patients, but photo-therapy,[1] as it is sometimes called, is a fairly new medium, needing systematic exploration in order to understand in what ways – and in what settings – photographs can help people.

In the first chapter, I explore the many meanings and implications behind photographs and how they are used by us all in our lives in different contexts. It is very simple to take a quick snapshot, but the complexities within the developed picture may be reflected on and pondered over for generations to come.

Chapter 2 illustrates some of the paradoxes and contradictions that are inherent in photographs. These stilled images can function as powerful reflectors of the ambivalence, confusion and inconsistencies that patients bring to therapy. They serve to highlight many of the themes within the patients's internal and external world. The exploration of this ambivalence often leads to some acceptance, resolution of inner conflict, and the self-understanding that so many of us seek.

Photographs can also be successfully incorporated into many different therapeutic styles and techniques. In Chapter 3, I shall give an overview of the various methods of photo-therapy, so that interested readers may make their own choice. Some therapists encourage a more active form of photo-therapy, with the patient engaged in the actual taking and making of the pictures. I have no formal photographic skills myself, and I am more interested in the meaning of the photograph than the process of taking it. I shall, therefore, mainly concentrate on the use of the patient's ready-made images in therapy.

I proceed further in Chapter 3 to an examination of some of the theories behind the use of photographs in therapy, showing how photographs may fit into the various therapeutic processes. The more detailed clinical material in the following chapter will illustrate some of these theoretical principles, providing an in-depth example of the use of photographs in therapy.

There follows, in Chapter 5, an exploration of the family album in a way that is intended to increase the therapist's skills in 'reading' photographs, in deciphering their secret language. There is also photographic illustration of how past experience influences present relationships. The theme is continued into the next chapter, which reveals how the family album can permit a new awareness of interactional patterns.

Chapter 7 describes the various groups of people who may gain from the therapeutic use of photographs, and explores how photographs can be adapted to different therapeutic styles and approaches.

Finally, Chapter 8 focuses on the relation between the photograph and the self, and the importance of the therapist's understanding of her own personal images. The purpose of this is to increase the therapist's self-knowledge and awareness through photographs, so that she can help others to do the same.

Some of the photographs in this book are posed by models, in order to protect the confidentiality of patients and their families. The reader will no doubt detect many anachronisms. In recreating the photographs, I have aimed for psychological accuracy in terms of feelings, atmosphere, expression and mood. I have not attempted to achieve historical correctness in relation to setting and dress.

My intention is to help readers of this book to look at photographs with a new and creative attitude, so that they will begin to see their therapeutic potential. So often, the manner in which we receive a photograph matches and reflects the shallow endeavour of the photographer. We, too, have a superficial approach as we peruse the countless 'happy' photographs of people responding to the mindless injunctions: 'Smile please. Say cheese. . . .' There is no conscious awareness of what the smiles might conceal.

Perhaps as you, the reader, leaf through this book, you will feel inspired to search out your own photographic memories. By maintaining an attitude of creativity, curiosity and openness, you may begin to discover what lies beyond the smile.

Acknowledgements

I should like to thank most sincerely the many patients who have so inspired my writing, and given me permission to tell their photographic stories.

I acknowledge with special gratitude my colleagues and friends Diana Lilley, Penny Grimshaw and Judy Rose for their support and encouragement. Sincere thanks also go to my parents for their help with research in Israel.

Without the assistance of photographer Yoka Jeffrey-Moeton, I should not have been able to recreate patients' photographs with such authentic realism. I am indebted to her for giving me so much of her time and for her most skilful contributions to this book. She has used her considerable abilities to copy the original photographs as far as possible, even when, in doing so, she was going against her own creative grain. Yoka is a professional photographer working near Manchester. She may be contacted at: Yoka Photography, 551, London Road, Stretton, Near Warrington, WA4 5PH.

Many of my friends and relatives have been invaluable as models, patiently posing, adopting difficult expressions; I do appreciate their considerable efforts on my behalf.

I am particularly grateful to Gloria Wade, Lisa Herzog and Janice Costa, all of whom have very considerably influenced my work with people who have been sexually abused.

I wish to acknowledge the social workers in both the fostering and adoption team at Trafford Social Services, and at the Hillsborough Centre in Liverpool. To those survivors of the Hillsborough disaster and their families, and to the survivors of the Holocaust who have shared their tragic stories with me, go my heartfelt thanks. I have also valued the help and instruction of Sister Karen Tate and her staff in Fox Ward, Sutton Hospital, Surrey.

I am grateful to the following for permission to reproduce material which has previously been published:

Charles (Mike) Doyle for lines from *Stonedancer* (Auckland University Press/Oxford University Press, NZ, 1976).

Macmillan London Ltd., for the poem 'Album', from *Frequencies* by R.S. Thomas (1978).

Margaret Newlin for the poem 'One for the Album'. First published in *Day of Sirens* (Carcanet Press), most recently in *Collected Poems 1963–1985* (Ardis, 1986. © Margaret Newlin).

Penguin Books Ltd., for photograph no. 20 from *A Vanished World* by Roman Vishniac (Allen Lane, 1983, © 1969, 1973, 1983 by Roman Vishniac, © 1947 by Schocken Books; renewal copyright 1975 by Roman Vishniac).

University of Pittsburgh Press for the poem 'Snapshot of Me as a Boy', reprinted from *Holding Patterns*, by Leonard Nathan (© 1982 Leonard Nathan).

My sincere appreciation goes to Colin Fox for his encouragement, enthusiasm and openness and for permitting me to publish aspects of his life story and some of his original photographs. Thanks also to Maggie Wilson, who has shared her photographs with me in an informative way, providing me with much valuable material.

I do not know how to express my gratitude to Joan Hargreaves, whose patience and wisdom have sustained me on my most difficult of journeys.

Above all, my deepest gratitude goes to Paul, my husband and my very best friend. He has supported me as I worked, and sometimes struggled, to put my ideas, my views, my very self, into the writing of this book. I could not have done so without his understanding and clear-sightedness, his unwavering encouragement and his love.

Chapter 1

Photographs in everyday life

'One for the Album'

> Who will recall
> That the red dog had fleas this summer
> And stank of the barn?
> That one child broke his brother's nose
> In August
> And the farm roof leaked?
> Those apples on the ground
> Hummed full of bees
> And smelled of rot.
> The camera never lies.
> It earmarks truth more ruthlessly than brush
> Making us climb forever there
> Over the white fence
> Under the apple tree
> Into the sunlit field.
> (Margaret Newlin, *Day of Sirens*)

Why do we like looking at photographs? Why do we often take such care with them, storing them and cherishing them, like treasures?

Before we take a more detailed look at the therapeutic use of photographs, it is necessary to understand their wider significance in our lives. Therapy is set against the backdrop of the world; it is important, therefore, to appreciate the wide range of cultural, social and popular attitudes to the camera and photographs and to consider the uses that we make of these in our day-to-day living. Therapists must develop and foster within themselves a keen awareness of these wider issues before beginning to contemplate the use of photographs in therapy. For photographs are not brought into therapy out of a void; they are taken out of life, and as such carry with them a whole set of issues and implications.

Let us take the time, therefore, to consider these broader themes in relation to photographs, thinking around them and beyond them. For it appears that, despite much careful preservation, the images on the whole tend to be viewed quite superficially, without thought for their deeper significance and meaning. With more profound examination, the pictures pose a multitude of questions.

THE PSYCHOLOGICAL SIGNIFICANCE OF PHOTOGRAPHS

Importance and appeal

The *Sun* newspaper once asked its readers: 'What would you grab first if the fire alarm went off?' One woman replied:

After the family were safe, I'd grab my photographs.
I can replace possessions, but not a lifetime of memories.

The appeal of the photograph is not restricted to any social class; its attraction is universal. The royal family obviously treasures its photographs as much as any family would. These, however, have an additional function; they simultaneously document the history of a family and that of a nation's monarchy.

Photographs perform useful practical functions in countless areas of life. They have for example, become an indispensable asset to the police, as identification, evidence and proof. They record events in newspapers and books, illustrating historical facts and giving information. They allow us to see the famous – and the infamous – at close quarters, giving pleasure to countless teenagers in the form of 'pop' posters – and bringing their heart-throbs right into the bedroom.

The fact that photographs 'have become an integral part of our lives' is confirmed by the results of a survey on photography conducted in June 1990 by a large photographic company. This nationwide survey revealed that:

We use photos to record those special moments and to underline our personal values.

96% of adults in the country love to keep photographs which capture their happy memories.

Eight out of ten of us hate to throw photographs away and almost half of us put them in albums.

There is a camera in 80% of British households.[1]

Thanks to the camera, it is relatively easy to express aspects of ourselves in pictures and to visually record selected features of our lives. The facility of photography is available to us all. Daguerre himself, who invented the first practicable photographic process in 1838, emphasised this point:

By this process, without any idea of drawing, without any knowledge of chemistry and physics, it will be possible to take in a few minutes the most detailed views, the most picturesque scenery, for the manipulation is simple and does not demand any special knowledge, only care and a little practice is needed to succeed perfectly. . . . This important discovery, capable of innumerable applications, will not only be of great interest to science, but it will also give a new impulse to the arts, and far from damaging those who practise them, it will prove a great boon to them. The leisured class will find it a most attractive occupation, and although the result is obtained by chemical means, the little work it entails will greatly please ladies.

(Trachtenberg 1980: 12–13)

Having been able to take a picture with such ease, we most often look forward to seeing the results of our photographic efforts. When photographs are collected from the processors, many people feel a sense of excitement at the prospect of seeing themselves, their families and friends, through the camera's eye.

The inhibited among us may wait for a private moment for perusal and possible censorship. The young and more open element often find it hard to keep the newly developed photographs in their envelope until they arrive home; they are excitedly opened on the spot.

For, in general, children love photographs. This love appears to relate to the delight in seeing themselves reflected. Catching a surprise glimpse of themselves in a mirror, a puddle – or a snapshot – is sure to produce squeals of joy. Children have a fascination with their own image, gazing enquiringly. They are also enthralled at the recognition of other family members on film. The reflection is confirming – of themselves and their identity. For children, the image can be a sign of the security of their place within the family and their world. From very early in life, this need to have oneself reflected is crucial to the development of the self:

Every child has a legitimate narcissistic need to be noticed, understood, taken seriously, and respected by his mother. In the first weeks and months of life he needs to have his mother at his disposal, must be able to use her and be mirrored by her. This is beautifully illustrated in one of Winnicott's images; the mother gazes at the baby in her arms, and the baby gazes at his mother's face and finds himself therein . . . provided that the mother is really looking at the unique, small, helpless being and not projecting her own introjects on to the child, nor her own expectations, fears and plans for the child. In that case, the child would not find himself in his mother's face but rather the mother's own predicaments. This child would remain without a mirror, and for the rest of his life would be seeking a mirror in vain.

(Miller 1987: 49)

Children need to be recognised as the unique and interesting small human beings that they are; *not* to be seen, to be ignored, or 'looked right through' is a most distressing experience for children and adults alike.

Reflected in the eyes of another, children can learn about themselves and their own identity. Thus, the sharing and recognition of their photographic image provides an exciting added bonus for children in the quest for identity and recognition; it validates them and their individuality, confirming both their separateness in the world and their relatedness to others. To be seen and admired in a photograph gives children a strengthening experience as they communicate the message 'This is me.'

The photograph provides us all, young and old, with an extra way of seeing and being seen; it helps us get ourselves noticed. As we select our photographs, we often show ourselves in the ways that we want to be seen, ways that match our desired internal image of ourselves. In showing the photograph, sharing it with others, we tend to watch their faces as they react to our image, checking out our impact on the other people, seeking their reflected acknowledgement and appreciation.

The effective therapist will be aware of this universal human need to have the self reflected, and will ensure that she helps the patient to have an experience in therapy of being heard, seen and understood in the eyes of the other.

Issues of control and rebellion

We want to keep our memories for all time; the very having of our photographs gives us a feeling that we have some control. This may be illusory, a denial, yet we cling tenaciously to our pictures. A recent television advertisement has as its theme song 'They can't take that away from me.' The film depicts a woman treasuring the photographic memory of a lost relationship.

We take such care of photographs because we know they connect us with our past; they are precious confirmation that we have existed, experienced, that we have been. They literally help us picture ourselves at different stages in our lives. The photographed moment, stretching out to infinity, lends us the time to absorb details at our leisure; we can control it in a way that gives us a feeling of power.

We may use photographs in any way we choose, employing fantasy and imagination. We can adore them, hate them, stick pins in them, display them, hide them, destroy or censor them. We can use them to deny or to confirm reality, to laugh or weep over, to preserve our desired image and maintain our fantasies.

The issue of control is often also present whilst the photographs are being taken. We can use the camera itself as a shield to avoid having to relate to people, or to intrude on their conversations. Photographing people gives the photographer the licence to control others by infantilising them and issuing orders:

Right, everyone, smile for the camera . . . Mabel, smile love, it may never happen. Elsie . . . please . . . stand still and move a little nearer to George. . . . Watch the birdie everybody!

We often react in a child-like way to these infantilising orders. Our behaviour whilst being photographed may be silly or absurd, as if we act out repressed urges. To some degree, this may be a reaction to feelings of self-consciousness and embarrassment, but the camera does also give some amongst us a freedom to relax our inhibitions and 'grab the limelight'.

Teenagers, especially, seize the opportunity to behave in a zany manner when faced with a camera. It is often a way of using their power to rebel against adults who want to control them into posing for a 'good' picture.

There are, however, people who hate being photographed. Perhaps they have unpleasant memories of being forced to pose as children, and now are using their adult choice to refuse such an experience. If they are 'captured' without permission, they may cover their face, turn away, protesting that they are 'camera shy'. A refusal to be photographed may also reflect a low self-image, a fear of seeing and being seen in a way that feels ultimately inescapable.

We can also use photographs to control others, especially through subjecting them to 'compulsory' looking. It is very difficult to decline an enthusiastic invitation to view someone's proudly proffered holiday snaps, for it would feel as though we were rejecting a part of them. There is a need in most of us to show our photographs to people who matter to us. It is good to have them admired and accepted, to have the approval of others and an unspoken confirmation that we are worth looking at.

Sometimes it is quite easy to appreciate another's photographs – they look interesting and one feels free enough with that person to browse through the snaps in an unconstrained way, without pressure. However, at other times, the showing of such holiday snaps is accompanied by a controlling, detailed and tedious narrative. Photographs reflect the person in more than one sense – the manner of presentation tells us much about their owner.

For the most part, other people's holiday snaps are just not as interesting as our own. Unless the presenter of the pictures is sensitive to this fact, the often reluctant onlookers are faced with a rather boring, repetitive set of holiday images – and one set looks very much like another.

But our own photographs are different – we have the memories; we can recollect the evocative smells, the warmth, the music, taste the food, reminisce over the new-found friends and reflect on the excitement of holiday romances. The pictures are treasured both as souvenirs and an important way of preserving our reminiscences.

Children on display

Often, photographs can become very special gifts, especially within the family. They may be presented in the form of cards, sent on special occasions, often expressly designed with a slot for the picture. School photographs are frequently sent to grandparents, who proudly exhibit their framed collections on pianos, mantelpieces and window-sills, delighting in their ever-increasing numbers. Perhaps the pictures stand as symbols of what they themselves have achieved and assurances that the family line will continue long after they have gone.

Furthermore, there is a curious truth in the fact that the photographs come to express their own reality, a larger than life quality, a sense of other-worldliness. They develop a value all of their own, an extra dimension. This point can be humorously illustrated by the following well-known Jewish joke:

> Mrs Levine, her face wreathed in proud smiles, was taking her infant daughter on her first outing. On the way, she encountered a neighbour who gushed over the baby.
> 'What a beautiful child!' the neighbour cried.
> Mrs Levine smiled delightedly. 'This is nothing,' she boasted. 'You should see her pictures!'

(Spalding 1969: 378)

Photographic mistakes and their relation to the unconscious

Not all photographs turn out as 'well' as Mrs Levine's. The family's camera is brought out to record all kinds of life events, and there are millions of photographs developed every year – with varying results.

For the seasoned amateur, it is sometimes difficult really to see what is framed by the camera's lens; often there is an anxiety to take the photograph quickly so we can carry on with life, for taking the posed picture momentarily stops everything. Photographer and subjects are stilled. In our haste to come back to life, to resume movement and action, we perhaps are not consciously aware of all we are seeing in one brief moment through the tiny viewfinder, with its capacity for instant time-seizure.

At times, maybe we try too hard to take a 'good' picture, with the result that the subjects tire, or adopt stilted poses. We may therefore be surprised that our pictures are quite different from how we had envisaged them at the moment of taking. Some give us untold pleasure, and emerge from the developers just as we would have wanted; others are disappointing 'failures'. We all have, at some time or another, taken photographs that are 'mistakes'. Sometimes, we may be frustrated because our pictures have not 'come out' as we consciously intended, or we may even be faced with

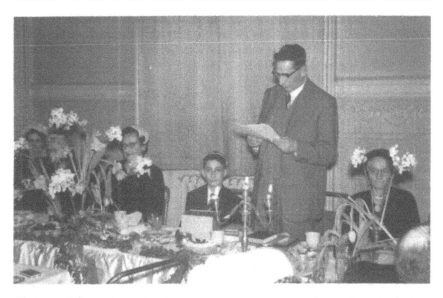

Photograph 1

blank prints. We discard them impatiently as if, momentarily, the sun in our life had been eclipsed, obscured. They feel like a waste, an opportunity missed, a kind of loss.

But what of the prints that are not blank, yet have not turned out as we expected? Can they, too, have meaning for us? I refer to the kind of photographs where father's head has been chopped off, where plants appear to be growing out of mother-in-law's hat (see Photograph 1), where wife is photographed at the zoo, with two zebras quietly copulating in the background.

Are these accidental 'mistakes'? Did the photographers really not see all that they were capturing on film? Or was there an unconscious desire to ridicule, have power, create humour? Perhaps this is a safe and subtle way of showing anger and rebelliousness, having the last laugh, getting one's own back, being care-less. Such errors may have significant unconscious meaning, and give us clues as to the hidden feelings towards the subjects. We may blame chance, or lack of skill, even a faulty camera or bad light for our mistakes. Yet we have made them, not the camera. This connects to the verbal 'accidents' we have, the slips of the tongue for which we may similarly deny responsibility, resisting seeing any deeper significance.

An example of such a photographic tongue-slip is described by Pierre Bourdieu:

The truly complete honeymoon is revealed by the couple photographed in front of the Eiffel Tower, because Paris is the Eiffel Tower, and because the true honeymoon is the honeymoon in Paris. One of the pictures in J.B.'s collection is bisected by the Eiffel Tower; at the bottom is J.B's wife. What seems to us an act of barbarism or barbarity is actually the perfect fulfilment of an intention.

(Bourdieu 1990: 36)

Subsequently, Bourdieu wonders: 'Conscious or unconscious?'

There are also occasions when photographs function as deliberate and somewhat mischievous mistakes. When on holiday in France, a friend was, apparently, snapping his two children, frolicking in the pool. But he obviously had frolics of a different kind in mind at the time, for the finished photograph reveals a woman wearing a topless bikini, behind the youngest child, and at the centre of the picture. The child in front of her poses for the camera, believing that the focus is on him. The older child, in the background, looks as though he has some suspicions about his father's true photographic motivation.

Another example of a deliberate photographic mistake: a friend's teenager, in the throes of considerable adolescent rebellion, was enjoying himself at an amusement park. By chance, he was asked by some strangers to photograph them as a family. When they had gone, the boy turned to me and said impishly: 'I cut their heads off. . . .' He had gleeful visions of their reaction when they saw the developed pictures; yet he was totally safe in the knowledge of his anonymity. This was mischief, power and control at a distance, a way of not doing what he had been asked, whilst appearing to do so.

In a more constructive way, 'accidental' mistakes can be used creatively. In his book about the experience of photography, Jeff Berner urges his readers to use their mistakes to produce another kind of image, another angle on the world. He stresses the importance of being able to capitalise on one's mistakes, see them as 'tools for deepening the range of creative possibility'. He suggests that these be explored and treasured for their artistic and impressionistic qualities. Berner quotes the example of one R. Buckminster Fuller who had blurred vision for the first four years of his life:

. . . his eyesight was so fuzzy that all he saw were large patterns. Faces were oval areas that spoke, houses were rectangular things with holes for walking in and out, and so forth. Before his vision 'handicap' was detected and corrected with glasses, he had time to learn the world as a complex of interrelated blurs of energy. So he did not begin his training as most of us do, with emphasis on getting details straight. Fuller grew up to become one of the most comprehensive and global thinkers of this century, and has spent his life teaching entire generations whole-systems thinking. His basic research is made up of details, but his mind remains omni-directional and highly conscious of the fact that the world is movement. One of his many books is titled *I seem to be a verb*.

(Berner 1975: 100)

These mistakes, then, our photographic spoonerisms and tongue-slips, need to be seen as potential areas of insight and learning about ourselves, from a different perspective. They may point to and emphasise the existence of the unconscious, and the contradictory messages and motivations that beset us as human beings. They can widen our view of the world.

CAMERA AND PHOTOGRAPH AS COMMUNICATION

Photographs constantly provide us with a vivid method of communication. Sometimes, concepts, feelings or visual experiences can be difficult to express linguistically and we may use photographs to enhance or replace our verbal description. It will be further shown in Chapter 7 how photographs may enhance communication for people who are unable to connect with others through words.

The taking of a photograph can also enhance communication, especially where there are language difficulties. Whilst on a touring holiday abroad, our coach stopped for a visit to a school. The children were eager to know about us, but they were also shy and uncomfortable. They spoke only a little English, and were reticent to use it. Something was needed to break the ice. Then, we decided to take a photograph. Immediately, the children grouped themselves for the camera (see Photograph 2). Responding excitedly, they posed happily for this universally familiar experience.

It had not been easy for the children to relate to us, a group of strangers, speaking in a foreign tongue. Yet note the connections made as they gestured at the lens, relaxing into communicative and friendly poses. Up to that point there had been little eye contact, but after the taking of the photograph, inhibitions lessened and communication was easier than before. As we photographed, they began to get in touch, literally and metaphorically – gesticulating, clowning and waving, all determinedly trying to get themselves in the picture.

Sharing the finished photographs with people from a different country also provides a way to diminish the language barrier, for they have a unique ability to cut across such restrictions on cross-cultural interaction.

Photographs can be seen as a powerful form of language: what is the nature of this language? How do photographs communicate their message? In what intricate ways can these soundless images speak to us? What are the limits of this language?

If we begin to consider these questions closely in relation to photographs, we may discover in them many new and interesting features. The pictures may soothe or shock, amuse or frighten, disgust, repel or attract

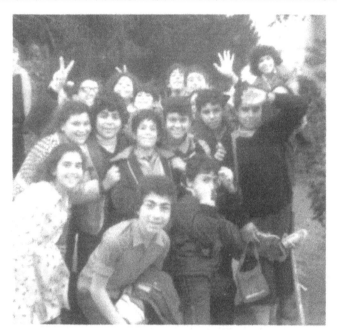

Photograph 2

us. They also ask questions that make us think and ponder. They give us a specifically descriptive kind of information, showing us more about the world in which we live. Exploring photographs with an open mind, using our powers of imagination, deduction and identification, we can receive strong and irrefutable messages from the visual images that remain uncluttered by the verbal.

To illustrate, let us examine Photograph 3 before we have the verbal explanation. Try to look at this picture in a new way, examining every part, perceiving the smallest nuances and expressions. In this way, it may actually be possible to perceive more than the actual photographer himself saw at the moment of taking the picture. We can view the moment at our leisure, as the photographer could not do, although, paradoxically, we are seeing less than he of that real moment in real time.

We see a man and a woman walking together. From their outward appearance, they look like fairly religious Jews, he with his beard, both with heads covered, most likely husband and wife. They look long married, perhaps they are into middle age. His collar and tie and formal buttoned-up coat could indicate that he has been at work; he carries a loosely tied parcel, she a torn basket. Her hands and face seem to indicate that she may have worked hard domestically, a homely, motherly woman. Her clothes look like those of an everyday housewife; perhaps she intended going to the market.

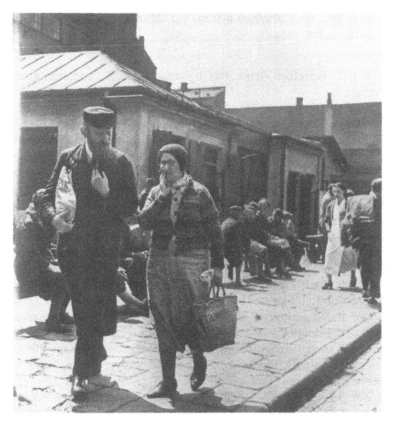

Photograph 3
© Roman Vishniac

The powerful impact of the photograph lies in the facial expressions, gestures and body-language of the two people. The woman looks shocked, stunned, as if the man is conveying some painful news to her. She seems to be gazing into space, thinking about what he is saying, perhaps beyond what he is saying, whilst listening intently to his words. The shape her mouth makes indicates her shock; the way her hand touches her face is perhaps an unconscious attempt to comfort herself.

Desmond Morris refers to this kind of behaviour as self-intimacy:

Self intimacies can be defined as movements that provide comfort because they are *unconsciously mimed acts of being touched by someone else.*

. . . There are many such ways in which we behave as if we were two people. The majority are only minor self-intimacies – little more than a fleeting touch – but the clue is there just the same: a little comfort is needed. The most common actions are those in which the hand comes up to touch the head.

(Morris 1986: 154–6)

We can tell, therefore, from this universal gesture, something of her consternation.

The man's hand points towards his chest – a gesture that says 'I' or 'me' – he is obviously talking about himself in some context. His face appears almost disbelieving and strained as he looks at his dismayed wife. A head taller than she at least, his steps are larger, but somehow her pace seems delayed and slowed by her emotional state. She is obviously his confidante, the two sharing some intensely awful news. They are not touching, but there is a feeling of closeness and involvement in their relationship.

There are other stories in the photograph. If we study it carefully, we can see that they are in a town or a city that is old and somewhat poor. The pavements are well worn, cracked and broken, the buildings shabby. Some of the people seem to be workers, going about their business. Perhaps it is their lunchbreak – the shadows are short and may indicate that it is around midday.

Two of those sitting on the bench in the background appear to be looking at the couple in the front of the picture, perhaps talking about them. If we let our imaginations wander, maybe we can hear the noises and smell the smells, feel the tension and worry that appears to be expressed in the faces.

We can glean much from the picture's silent communication. Yet, once we have such information from the photograph, there will remain un-answered questions. Whilst the photograph has in many ways spoken for itself, there are, inevitably, explanations it cannot give. We need some narrative to clarify and confirm the visual messages.

Here, then, are the facts the photograph cannot tell us: it was taken in the Warsaw Ghetto by Roman Vishniac in 1937. He explained that after taking it, he asked the couple about their problem:

The husband told me that he had just been fired from his job as manager of his firm. The owner had been well satisfied with him for twenty years, but that morning three men came to the office to check whether any Jews were employed there. He was immediately dismissed, with no compensation, no hope of another job. The good life was over in an instant.

(Vishniac 1983)

A photograph can also express a powerful message when it is used in a metaphorical way. Metaphor has been described as 'transfer of meaning' (Ortony 1975: 45) and is a vivid and indispensable method of communicating through images and symbols. We can use photographs to express our thoughts and feelings metaphorically. To understand metaphor, however, one has to be able to use imagination creatively and to think in a symbolic way. Where this is possible, there is an intensity of communication through a photographic metaphor that provides us with vivid, instantaneous and immediate expression.

After the disaster at the Hillsborough football ground in Sheffield in 1989, a young boy found he was unable to talk to social workers about his ordeal. He was given magazines to look through, in the hope of helping him find suitable images through which he might be able to communicate. After some time, he chose a picture of a headless, bloody chicken to begin to express some of his feelings.

He could not express this verbally, for language had become inhibiting; the metaphorical image helped free him. He was in fact saying: 'This photograph exactly sums up the way I feel.'

Dramatic pictures of the floral tributes laid out on the pitch at Hillsborough became metaphors for all the loss of life. These photographs were intensely meaningful to the families and survivors: they symbolised so much about the fragility of life and the need to remember and pay tribute. We can also create pictures with the camera that metaphorically express our inner 'landscape'. A description of such a photograph will be found in Chapter 8.

TIME AND THE PHOTOGRAPH

Photographs provide a way of keeping visual recollections of the past safe from the dulling grasp of time; so we store them with care, cherishing them.

For photography preserves the fleeting moment forever. Looking back through time to a single frozen instant, we are inevitably confronted with the passing years, the transience of our lives. Without the camera, these moments would have been unregistered, unrecorded, erased, like footprints in the sand obliterated for all time by the relentless surge of the sea. But now we may look back, and ponder. We have the facility to compare past and present. We can stand these side by side, as it were, to measure the differences and contrasts and to discover the connections.

We may trace the patterns and recurrences of life in our photographs. As we wonder at the coincidences, similarities and parallels, we witness history repeating itself right in front of us.

Whilst the single photographed moment may be fleeting, it is not free-floating, it fits into a continuous flow in time. It is a second's flash in a multi-coloured life-story that has specificity of meaning, a life-theme that develops up to and after the photographic moment.

Many religious and philosophical beliefs support the view that life repeats itself over and over again, either in a circular or spiral pattern. Whether or not we accept these beliefs, the concept is interesting in relation to the study of photographs.

It encourages us to contemplate the recurrences in our own lives and perhaps to explore which patterns can be changed, once they are brought to consciousness, and which are beyond our control. The camera slices out moments in the circle of time and preserves them. In a series of captured photographic moments, we may recognise and trace returning themes and images. Before us, for perpetual contemplation, is the recurrence of the seasons and the endless cycle of births, marriages and deaths. We may discover there family resemblances, modes of behaviour and relationships that repeat themselves in a seemingly cyclical manner.

Like grand designs, these patterns continue, intertwining and spiralling through the generations as they weave their repetitive track through time. These ways of being and relating are passed down over the years and persist into the future; if we take heed of what the photograph is mirroring for us, we may learn to understand and perhaps change negative behaviour patterns.

Our albums of pictures may at one level be material, tangible legacies from the past, bringing it vividly alive in the present. At another level, they can reveal to us something of our inner, unconscious inheritance in terms of personal patterns and family systems. They can do this by showing us the past in the present, so that we can make connections which may help us in the future. In Chapter 5, we shall see examples of such patterns from the family album.

Whilst reflecting on these repeating themes, we are faced in our photographs with the ghosts of the past, present, and perhaps with portents of the future. In perusing them, we can experience time in an almost magical way, freed from the constraints of the 'now'. This power of the photograph to transcend time itself seems almost surrealistic, for different time phases are linked and encapsulated, creating a feeling of 'all time'. This means that the photograph can serve both as an aid to memory and a facilitator of present awareness; past and present are thrown into relief.

In a curious way, the photograph is also like a pointer to the future, a sign, making implications about possible consequences. This multi-functional aspect is nowhere better illustrated than in the grim photographic images of the Holocaust, variously taken by the Nazis, by the victims themselves, survivors and underground photographers. Here photographs do indeed serve simultaneously as memories and prophecies, omens for the future.

These distressing memorials immediately confront us with the past, starkly emphasising the link between photography and death.

Before our eyes is 'that rather terrible thing which there is in every photograph: the return of the dead' (Barthes 1988: 9).

Implicit in the solemn images of the Holocaust are also cautionary signs, portentous predictors of sinister future possibilities. If we see beyond the monochromatic veneer of the picture, like crystal gazers, we may discover the latent messages within.

Barthes has said of photography: 'It is a prophecy in reverse: like Cassandra, but eyes fixed on the past . . .' (Barthes 1988: 87).

Where Holocaust photographs are concerned, this prophecy moves multi-directionally. Photography becomes a prescient medium that simultaneously anticipates in the future what it documents in the past. It also has implications for the present. However, such warnings can only become activated if we choose to look, to note their messages and to learn from them.

The photograph and eternity

In a slightly different, though related vein, time may be experienced as eternal in the context of photographs, in a mystical way. It would appear that photographs can have a higher function than merely to show the course of history repeating itself. They can have a reconstructive role, and the result of this may reveal an uncanny spiritual dimension.

An example of this may be seen in the vivid and powerful experience of Hanna Abells, who was archivist at Yad Vashem, Jerusalem, for fifteen years prior to her retirement. Yad Vashem is a memorial place and museum of the Holocaust and many relatives of the dead visit there to discover evidence of their lost loved ones, or to record their names or photographs. Survivors have brought testimonies to Hanna to corroborate the photographic evidence.

Hanna described the effect of continual long-term exposure to Holocaust photographs. During her years at the Memorial Centre she studied and rearranged the whole of the photographic archives several times. The incredible impact of this photographic collection on Hanna is that, although she was never in a concentration camp herself, she actually feels that she has been there. She relates:

> It's as though I were there because I can tell you everything – I have visual memories without ever having been there. I worked with the survivors first, then I heard their testimonies. As they spoke, about Maidenek, or Auschwitz, for example, I could picture it. I could see exactly what they were describing. It feels like it is something to do with the rabbinical injunction that we strive to accomplish: in every generation people should feel as if the past is shared, has happened to us . . . as if we experience again what has happened to our ancestors.

Hanna is referring to a pronouncement that 'In every generation, every Jew must feel as if he himself came out of Egypt' (Deuteronomy 6.23).

Hanna has felt her experiences to be more than the result of prolonged and constant exposure to the photographs. Spiritually, she has lived through the horrors with the victims in some intangible and mystical way. The photographs have in fact replaced and transcended memory for her and enabled a completely felt reanimation of the past. Through them, Hanna does more than identify with the victims; it is as if she is transformed into them, in a different time, a different place, within the context of eternal time. The photographs have helped her to become acutely aware of the eternity which encloses every moment; each moment then becomes a part of a whole, lasting reality.

PHOTOGRAPH AS MAGIC

The magical, mystical quality of the camera implies that it possesses a power greater than itself. Indeed, many primitive peoples refuse to be photographed, fearing that they will be robbed of their soul by the camera's sorcery and be bewitched by its voodoo. The images it produces are seen as having an influence far beyond themselves, able to weave and cast magic spells. They are not just pictures of a person, but a part of that person imbued with his/her spirit. If they fall into the wrong hands, they can be used to harm or even kill the person they represent.

In certain parts of the world today where magic is still practised, photographs have been seen as having magical powers. People have therefore tried to avoid letting their photograph fall into enemy hands, where they might be used for evil ends. Photographs have been used in the practice of witchcraft, in much the same way as the voodoo dolls or puppets are used. These images 'become' the intended victim in the mind of the person practising witchcraft, and spells and rituals are performed upon them. The photograph may also have been attached to the doll, creating a vividly personalised symbol on which to work for good or ill.

There are some powerful superstitions that have become attached to photographs. Some people still believe that having their photograph taken will bring bad luck upon them. *The Encyclopaedia of Superstitions* describes some of these fears:

> If an engaged couple are photographed together, something will happen to prevent the marriage. In the Transactions of the Devonshire Association (Vol. 90, 1958) it is recorded that in March of that year, two Devonshire football teams refused to allow a Press photographer to take a picture of them before the game on the grounds that it was very unlucky to be photographed before a match.
>
> (Radford and Radford 1961: 263)

This view of the photograph as magical is, indeed, still prevalent today. Susan Sontag refers to an aspect of this attitude in discussing the photograph as a good luck charm or talisman:

> The lover's photograph hidden in a married woman's wallet . . . the snapshots of a cab driver's children clipped to the visor . . . such

talismanic uses of photographs express a feeling both sentimental and implicitly magical: they are attempts to contact or lay claim to another reality.

(Sontag 1987: 16)

CAN THE CAMERA LIE? REALITY AND THE PHOTOGRAPH

More and more questions emerge. What of the issue of reality and the photograph? Can we trust them to tell us the truth simply because they are the result of a technical process?

We do tend to rely on photographic truth in order really to see past events for ourselves. We are able to trust the permanently visible, whilst we can doubt memory or verbal descriptions. Both Milgram and Sontag stress this point:

> For the camera provides a mechanical and exhaustive rendering of visual surfaces, within the range of its technical capacities. This directness and infinite inclusiveness confer on photographs a high degree of credibility. We are more likely to believe that an object depicted in a photograph really existed than, say, an object depicted in a painting.
>
> (Milgram 1977: 342)

> . . . a photograph is not only an image (as a painting is an image), an interpretation of the real; it is also a trace, something directly stencilled off the real, like a footprint or death mask.
>
> (Sontag 1987: 154)

Thus, photographs can be used as firm evidence that will be valid in a court of law, with verbal corroboration. They may clearly document history, and can inform and educate. They come to represent the real and the true, and are seen as factual proof, confirmation that events occurred and people existed.

However, in themselves, photographs possess no definite or precise meaning. In order to be reliable as evidence, and to combat the elements of selectivity and reductionism, they need to be authenticated and correctly identified. They testify only to a happening.

As Barthes has said: 'Photography never lies; or rather it can lie as to the meaning of the thing, being by nature *tendentious*, never as to its existence. . . . Every photograph is a certificate of presence' (Barthes 1988: 87).

Therefore, whilst this 'presence' is irrefutable, its meaning and significance can be misinterpreted; it is relatively easy to look at a picture and make fictional assumptions about it. These are perhaps more related to our own projections than to any kind of objective reality.

A photograph may also give us a false and unreal impression because of its reductiveness, or because of the intention of the photographer, the poor quality of the camera or dubious photographic skills. Furthermore, photographs can very easily be doctored: 'While photographs may not lie, liars may photograph.'[2] They have long been tools of propaganda and deception, because the medium and its meaning are so manipulable. Even when the intention is a fairly honest one, fabrications may still be used in terms of the photograph. Techniques of manipulation are often used in advertising, for instance, where scenarios may be staged to appear convincingly real. The camera, like many other instruments, can serve the purposes of humanity in either a truthful or dishonest way, according to the intentions of its user.

The truth may thus be deliberately hidden, or the very nature and limitations of photography itself can hide and distort the truth. Whilst photography makes implications about other phases of time, it cannot record every moment, therefore it is by its nature selective. The whole of one's life and growth cannot be photographed; human life is simply too long to be captured on film in its entirety. One cannot show a human being growing day by day, like a flower, and speed it up to make a full life-story in pictures.

The photograph is inevitably selective, in that it has a frame. Life on film is outlined, bordered, edged, whereas the real world does not have edges. It is infinite. The camera inescapably encloses and delineates, creating a constructed reality. It is conditioned, restricted by its technicality. Inevitably then, photography has to be an endeavour that is defined and somewhat determined by these limitations and human bias and selectivity.

In earlier days of photography, camera users were urged to photograph only in the sun, never in the shade. We have, however, continued to pose and smile in the sun for the camera; thus we create myths about the good, the happy – a one-sided picture.

There are yet more factors that will contribute to this reductionism. The attitude of the photographer, either conscious or unconscious, must be taken into account. He or she will certainly be influenced by personal ways of seeing the world and the people in it. This will inevitably affect the finished result. It is, however, most often difficult to detect from the actual photograph the attitudes behind the taking and the relationship between photographer and subject. We may perceive different features which could be assumed to indicate something of the photograph's intentions; however, these may be the viewer's own projections onto the photograph. They may also be attributed to varying photographic skills and camera quality.

THE OTHER SIDE OF THE PICTURE: THE WOUNDING IMAGE

Photographers may have many reasons for taking their photographs. They may be motivated by a desire to capture the essence of things, to record truth, beauty and life in general; to tell a story, to communicate a feeling or an opinion. On the other hand, they may be driven by greed, power or a desire to exploit and damage. The great paradox inherent in photography is that, whilst the camera may be used in many positive ways, photography can become an aggressive act.

Used intrusively, the camera can represent a violation and abuse of privacy. The vocabulary of the photographer vividly reflects this idea of the camera as a weapon. Scanning through various photographic magazines, I pinpointed the following words, phrases and extracts:

> The CP-9AF is packed with creative features such as a built-in Interval Timer to *capture* the magic of an opening flower or setting sun. With Catch-in Focus you can automatically *trigger* the shutter to freeze your subject . . .
>
> (Chinon advert)

One magazine mentions 'powerful and arresting images', and recommends 'a head shot, tightly cropped'. An advertisement for camera film tells us: 'Your shooting is only as good as your ammunition'. Words like 'exposure', 'zoom', 'flash', 'frame', 'snap', 'load', 'shoot', 'close-up', further convey this sense of aggression. 'Taking' a photograph suggests that we actually rob the subject of some kind of essence or image, which is exactly what some people fear from the camera. This invasive use has been rationalised in terms of the need for news or for reasons of historical evidence, as if the end always justified the means.

At the turn of the century, photographers sought to photograph the lives and customs of the Hopi Indians. Some used their cameras with respect, whilst others:

> . . . abused their privileges and felt compelled to photograph forbidden subjects. Such illicit photography was probably tied both to curiosity and a conviction that Hopi traditions must be recorded for posterity, whether or not the Hopi people agreed. Photographs taken inside Kiras (underground ceremonial chambers) are most notable examples of this abuse. Secretive field methods, however, were used in many other situations, sometimes to record 'unusual' subject matter, other times to capture a 'candid' effect.
>
> (Masayesva and Younger 1984: 21)

The taking of photographs without the permission of the subject represents a gross violation of liberty, privacy and choice. Recording such material on camera, and then showing it to the world, for personal gain or satisfaction, or for propaganda purposes, is a flagrant infringement of human rights.

(There must, however, be a differentiation between this abusive use of the camera and the taking of photographs in order to inform the world about sensitive issues or major disasters. The latter fulfils a very necessary function and is quite different from taking photographs for abusive reasons. The paradox here is that very similar, or even identical photographs may be taken – with very different motives.)

The Nazis abusively photographed the dead and dying victims of their own horrendous crimes. Sometimes they photographed them just prior to murdering them; this is bestiality at its most voyeuristic. Often, such pictures were proudly sent home to relatives by the Nazis. Regarded as personal 'souvenirs', these were on occasion assembled in neat albums, macabre travesties of the traditional family album.

One such collection, compiled by SS Officer Kurt Franz, was entitled 'The Best Years of My Life'. This is an extreme and viciously abusive use of the camera as weapon; yet still in society today, the camera is used in ways that are hurtful and distressing.

There has been much controversy about the intrusiveness and manipulative behaviour of the press and press photographers. Some photographs are deliberately taken with the intention of lying. Others have been doctored. The fact that photographs are manipulable has been exploited over the years in areas like advertising and propaganda.

Without caption, explanation or context, photographs can, of course, be interpreted in several different ways and ascribed many meanings. Yet even a caption, however historically and contextually precise, may influence us by its inescapable subjectivity. In unscrupulous hands, the context and meaning of photographs can be manoeuvred, twisted and altered to suit various purposes. Mischief and scandal have been created by such distortions, causing much distress to those targeted.

In December 1990, the *Sun* newspaper was censured by the Press Council for intruding on the Prince of Wales and Lady Romsey. They published pictures of them .together during the summer and made an 'outrageous' insinuation.

The picture showed the two on its front page, in Majorca, the Prince with his arm round Lady Romsey. The headline was: 'Prince hugs his old flame', and the caption said: 'Royal snuggle . . . Charles, wearing white bathing trunks, cuddles gorgeous Penny at the remote villa.'

The photograph itself, open to any kind of misinterpretation, was used to imply that the two were more than friends. In fact, Lady Romsey had just confided to Prince Charles that her young daughter had cancer.

The taking of photographs of the famous and of royalty, without their consent, is often seen as justifiable in terms of 'news'. The front page of the *Sunday Sport*, 4 March 1990, proudly displays a photograph of injured actor Gorden Kaye, lying in hospital. The caption beneath states: 'SNATCHED – photos of Gorden taken without his consent.'

The headline reads:

Bedside shots taken without consent
TV STAR RENE . . . PHOTOS HE TRIED TO BAN

Legal action taken over the illicit pictures resulted in permission being granted to publish them by the High Court, on condition that the paper stated that the photographs were taken without the permission of the subject.

The paper seems to further add to its abuse of the actor by proudly proclaiming this fact as a sort of triumph or achievement on its part:

AMAZING SNEAK PICTURES!

During and after human disasters, there have been examples of photographers bringing us desperate and desolate pictures; one may wonder in some cases why they were not rather putting their energies into helping their suffering 'subjects'. Yet, there is a need for press photography to inform, to tell the world, to give pictorial evidence of such disasters. There is an eternal dilemma here, raising much anxious debate and involving several complicated and paradoxical issues.

Where is the line to be drawn between taking a photograph to inform and to promote understanding, and taking one for selfish and intrusive motives? Do the resulting pictures increase awareness and understanding or do they actually desensitise the viewer towards violence and pain?

These questions are most starkly relevant in relation to the Hillsborough football disaster. There is video evidence, as well as survivors' stories, about press photographers rushing through the panicking crowds to stand over the bodies of the dead and dying, in order to obtain 'scoop' photographs. The horrific results of their efforts were splashed across many front pages the following day. Clearly recognisable individuals were photographed in close-up, in their last, agonising, dying moments. As they were being crushed to death against the railings by the helplessly surging crowd, their excruciating torment was photographed for all to see.

After the publication of these photographs, there was a Press Council enquiry. It concluded that publication of those pictures of the Hillsborough disaster which had been taken from a distance, was justifiable: 'It is the job of newspapers to report news including tragedy and horror and sometimes to awaken public conscience or determination that tragedy shall not be repeated.' However, where close-up photographs of the dead and dying were concerned, 'the intrusion into personal agony and grief was too gross to be justifiable'.

There is an expectation that individual photographers and newspaper editors will be aware of these matters of conscience in relation to pictures of pain and disaster. Unfortunately, this is not always the case, and some newspaper photographs continue to cause pain, or to be used for purposes of sensationalism.

We have seen in this chapter something of the significance of photographs, their influence and psychological impact on the lives of all of us. There has been exploration of the motives behind the taking, sharing and keeping of photographs, together with their potential to teach and inform us.

Finally, we have examined their power in our world, and how they are utilised in many different ways. It has been shown that they can be taken with motives of greed and used to devastating effect. Pornographers also take pictures that depersonalise and degrade, perpetuating the use of the camera as weapon, invader, penetrative intruder. But these issues are part of another story.

Suffice it to say that, as with any kind of power, we can choose to use the photographic image in our lives for destructive ends, or with good intent, for healing. The photograph can also bring great joy and harmony into our lives, an appreciation of beauty and colour, a way of meeting others in a mutual experience of telling and remembering. Where photographs are concerned, paradoxes and contradictions such as this abound. Within the individual photograph itself, opposites are joined in visual symmetry, though these are barely discernible to the superficial eye. In the following chapter, it will be demonstrated how important is the deeper study of such paradoxes in our photographs, in order that we may learn to use them therapeutically and to enhance our awareness of self and other.

Chapter 2

'I am here, I am there'

Paradoxes, contradictions and ambiguities within the photograph

'Album'

My father is dead.
I who am look at him
Who is not, as once he
Went looking for me
in the woman who was.

There are pictures of the two of them, no
need of a third, hand
in hand, hearts willing
to be one but not
three.

What does it mean
life? I am here I am
there. Look! Suddenly
the young tool in their hands
for hurting one another.

And the camera says:
Smile; there is no wound
time gives that is not bandaged
by time. And so do the
three of them at me who weep.
                    (R.S. Thomas, *Frequencies*)

Photographs reflect life in all its infinite variety. The human condition, with its uncertainties and ambivalence, is expressed potently through the camera's eye. Within the photograph we will discover graphic evidence of such ambiguities, vivid and meaningful images of contradictory realities.

Reconciling these opposites and coming to terms with their existence within the self is an essential factor in the achievement of psychological health. Photographs can provide us with a powerful way of understanding and working through the paradoxes and incongruities that beset us daily, internally and externally.

The dictionary defines paradox as 'a statement seemingly contradictory or absurd, though possibly well-founded or essentially true'.[1] Therapists can learn much from the study of the essential paradoxical truths to be found in a photographic statement. Understanding the concept of paradox is highly relevant to both therapy and the photograph, because each in its own way reflects the ambivalence and confusions of life.

Whilst we wrestle with life's contradictions, grappling with its inconsistencies, the photograph silently mirrors them, seemingly without disharmony. It displays them in such clever reconciliation, that often the conflicting aspects escape our conscious awareness and we miss the paradoxes within.

Before I examine in some detail the use of photographs in therapy, it is pertinent in this chapter to concentrate the reader's attention on such photographic paradoxes. Unless there is a keen awareness of these, there will be limitations on the use of the photograph as an adjunct to therapy.

A PLETHORA OF PHOTOGRAPHIC PARADOXES

'Neither black nor white, but both . . .'

If we take the time to 'read' photographs on more than one level, they can help us to explore the hitherto unknown opposites within ourselves. Photographs confront us with paradoxes in an immediate way, displaying them before our very eyes, in stark monochrome or flagrant colour. Perhaps they can, paradoxically, say more than words, because of this visual dimension.

The inevitable limitations of language are clearly explained in relation to Zen Buddhism:

> The symbols we use in language can become a barrier when they are confused with what is out there and inside here. Life is infinitely more complex and beautiful than any of our words and sentences allow. We cannot easily describe forces moving off in different directions. What words do we use when things are neither true nor untrue, neither black nor white, but both?
>
> Words stumble after capturing the essence of life which is continuously changing shape, always on the move. They try to define the indefinable. They resemble a sports commentator on the radio continuously describing a football game which has since changed. What we call paradoxes occur when the limits of sentences to describe several contradictory processes are reached. The Zen masters were too practical, too rooted in the earth to get caught in those sticky nets.
>
> (Brandon 1976: 18–19)

'Neither true nor untrue, neither black nor white, but both' – these are exactly the paradoxes within the photograph. They can surely help us to move outside our narrow frame of reference. Like the Zen masters, we may begin to think beyond the contradictions and open them out into possibilities for growth and change. We may thus be stimulated by them to ask questions, to venture further.

At this point, then, we may begin to wonder: what are the kinds of paradoxes to be found in a photograph? How does the identification of these help to expand our view, to think more holistically, see the complete, contradictory picture? How can they help to combat denial, widen our perceptions? What sort of paradoxes do therapists need to be aware of when contemplating working with photographs? What are the links between the paradoxes within the photograph and those within the therapy situation?

Let us now take a closer look at some of the many paradoxes within the photograph, exploring them with a view to increasing our awareness of the complexities beneath the image. As these paradoxes are revealed, it will become increasingly clear how potentially valuable will be their contribution to the process of therapy. It will also become evident how important is the therapist's shrewd understanding of their power and complexity.

The 'photographic look' and other camera tricks

When we look at a photograph, we see, and we do not see, and the people in the photograph look back at us, smiling, yet they are neither seeing us nor looking at us. Barthes calls this the 'photographic look', sometimes seen in life, and describes it in the eyes of boy in a cafe: 'I then had the certainty that he was *looking at me* without however being sure that he was *seeing me*: an inconceivable distortion: how can we look without seeing?' (Barthes 1988: 111).

In the poem 'Album', the poet points out that the photograph of himself as a child with his parents shows the three of them looking at him, looking at the photograph. The extra paradox here, is that the child poet is looking at *himself*, yet once again, there is the looking without seeing (see Photograph 4 for an example of such 'photographic looks').

Equally, as we look at a photograph, we can hear without hearing, smell without smelling, touch without touching, even taste without tasting. Advertisers depend on the power of our imaginations to savour the smell and flavour of photographed food and feel the softness of the puppy in the famous toilet roll advertisement. We may touch the picture of our loved one, hold him or her in our hand, but we are not touching or holding the person at all. Similarly, a picture may depict frenetic, whirling movement, as in dancing, or other intense physical activity. Yet the photograph is motionless.

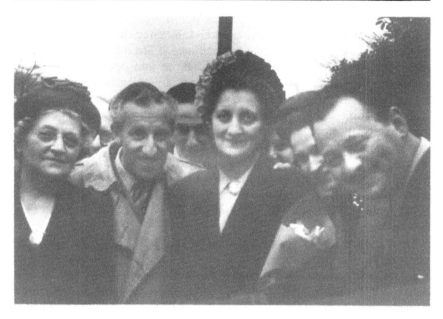

Photograph 4

Fantasy and reality

These two levels of experience are mingled in the photograph in a way that may confuse and fascinate; often they are both interwoven and the uncertainty exploited in order to sell a product, or for the purposes of humour.

The following stand up comic's joke, makes use of the ease with which fantasy and reality can be muddled in a photograph:

> Comedian, with an object in his hands covered with a black cloth:
> 'Ladies and gentlemen, I'd now like to show you a picture of the famous escapologist, Houdini . . .'
> (pulls off cover, and is holding an empty frame)
> '. . . Well look at that, he's got away again!'
>
> (Tommy Cooper)

Dangerously large . . . or safely small?

The photograph also plays tricks with dimension. We may perceive a man in a photograph as tall, even immense in size, yet there he is, no taller than an inch. Furthermore, the perception of great size may not always relate to physical dimensions.

Sometimes, a person of average height may seem monstrous in size in a photograph, because he or she has a massive emotional impact on the viewer. This often happens when patients are looking at photographs of parents in therapy. The photograph is a symbol; at times, however, it transcends the symbolic and appears, within the mind, to extend into the real. Yet, simultaneously, there is the firm knowledge that in reality it is safe and familiar, having no substantial power to harm. It may thus help patients in therapy to venture into the less certain level of the unconscious, and the insecure world of childhood fears and feelings.

Meaning and no meaning

Yet can it be that this is no more than a piece of printed card, or that the photograph is no symbol at all, but merely an image, a superficial affair, material for idle chat?

For some, it is indeed heavily symbolic, for others, it is not so. We may perceive it on two levels. On a factual level the photograph may be seen as merely an image, an arrangement of light, shade and shape on a flat surface, an effective way of visually representing a reality. At a deeper level, this same picture can be endowed with meaning. It can be used as a metaphor for many inner feelings and is rich in significance.

As we have seen in Chapter 1, photographs need a narrative to explain their meaning, yet they can stand on their own. Thus they are both meaningful and meaningless.

Public and personal

An important additional paradox connected with the photograph and meaning resides in the fact that it can be both public and personal, general and specific. A personal photograph of close relatives serves as a way of delineating the family for the family, defining and describing the members within it. To an outsider, however, it is quite difficult to recognise the members of a family through an unknown photograph. One can look for resemblances, but it will be difficult to identify members of the family in any definitive way.

Yet a most personal and especially significant photograph, full of hidden, distinctive family features, when viewed by a stranger, can still have meaning. This will be necessarily different from the personal meaning.

When a photograph, especially one depicting human suffering, is anonymous and is not accompanied by caption, narrative or explanation, a change occurs in the way it is regarded. Its meaning expands and generalises, the images widen into archetypal symbols; it becomes a part of the universal archives of human affliction. Individual experience is transcended. In Jungian terms, we can relate to the now universal images because they reflect those in the 'collective unconscious', a shared store of symbols that is deeply imprinted in our psyche, common to us all (Jung 1978: 41).

There is a shift of meaning, a redefiniton and reshaping in terms of context and significance, as fuller and more extensive interpretations evolve and unfold. Yet the precise and detailed personal meanings of the picture still have relevance; they stand now alongside the general, which reflects them.

An example of such a photograph would be that of the naked little girl in Vietnam running screaming from her village after a horrendous napalm attack. This is a child we all know – and can picture – and yet we do not know her personally; we cannot have the same kind of feelings as we would if she were a part of our family. We feel for her pain, her fear and her helplessness. Her picture has also come to symbolise the acute terror and pointlessness of such atrocities, and the destructiveness of war.

There are important links to and reflections of this photographic paradox in the therapy situation. A patient's problems are specifically personal to him or her in a way that is unique in terms of their content and detail. Yet these problems will inevitably reflect the whole human condition and the therapist will recognise countless universal themes in her patient's story.

As a therapist, I can identify with the aspects that I recognise in another's photographs – and can enquire about those I do not. As I look at other people's photographs, I am doing something that is familiar to me – I am used to looking at and sharing such things, they are a part of my world, too. Whilst being careful not to over-identify, there are bound to be themes in their pictures that I can recognise. I too know what it is like to go on holiday, to have a party, to hold a new baby.

At the same time, I observe that there are considerable differences in another person's pictures. I see there a collection of people I have never met who remain unaware that I, this stanger from a future time, will be gazing questioningly into their lives. Therefore – whilst we are brought closer by the sharing and the recognition of this familiar activity – the distance and differences between us are also emphasised.

Power and powerlessness

The issue of control is an interesting and contradictory one in relation to the photograph. We can feel in control of people when their photograph is in our possession. We can do anything to the picture – and yet we have no power over those people through the photograph, we affect them not at all.

Whilst some people do feel controlling and powerful in relation to their photographs, others fear that they will be controlled; they have a strong sense of the power of the photograph to disturb them and almost come alive before their very eyes. Even though the photograph is in itself limited, it is unlimited in terms of what it can symbolise for patients. The photograph can represent anything they want. In fantasy, they can use the picture in a myriad of ways; it becomes remarkably meaningful.

Thus, when photographs are used in therapy, their possible forceful effects on the patient should never be underestimated; they need to be treated with care and caution. For the emotions triggered by the images are conflicting and paradoxical; initially they can precipitate intense confusion, as internal inconsistencies and ambivalent feelings become more apparent. In this way, the photograph may be seen as unsafe and menacing.

On another level, of course, it has no power at all, other than that which is projected onto it. It is merely a piece of printed paper, safe and harmless, innocuous enough.

The fear is an internal one, although it feels like an external threat, some kind of spectre coming to haunt and torment. Sometimes, people talk to photographs without realising that they are, in fact, addressing aspects of themselves.

The reflexive paradox

But surely it is impossible to both be ourselves and talk to ourselves? This is the paradox of self-reference and it applies equally to the photograph, which creates its own paradoxes. A picture cannot picture itself, someone else has to picture it:

A picture, one might remind oneself, cannot depict itself because an image cannot be 'of' itself; it has, so to speak, to face outwards and be 'of' things other than itself.

(Champlin 1988: 123)

Thus, a painting by René Magritte[2] shows an image of a pipe, with the caption: 'Ceci n'est pas une pipe'.

The paradox of self-reference is relevant to patients in therapy who, for example, may be talking to mother in a photograph but they are actually talking to a part of themselves that has absorbed an image of mother. However, paradoxically, at one level, in terms of the photograph, they are also talking to mother. Using the photograph in this way provides the therapist with an excellent medium through which to help patients get in touch with the various parts of their personality, and it also helps them recognise and identify projections and assumptions.

For example, the middle-aged man who rebukes his strict father in a photograph for 'making' him feel shame amd guilt all his life, is, in part, addressing a facet of his own personality. Long after his childhood days, he is reacting to an internalised version of his father, now incorporated into his own self. This is a part of him that is strict and rigid with himself, that cannot let go of the old unpleasant yet familiar ways of being. He perceives internal feelings as external, an unconscious way of avoiding confrontation with difficult aspects of the self.

Analogous to this is the phrase 'I don't know myself'; this is similarly paradoxical.

Another reflexive paradox, this time in connection with the camera, can again be seen in the poem, 'Album':

And the camera says:
Smile;

Of course, the camera does not say this, nor does it take the picture, although we often refer to it as though it does. Frequently, actions are attributed to objects or people in ways that sound quite ludicrous when analysed. The camera is given a power beyond itself, endowed with human abilities to take photographs spontaneously.

The strange and the familiar

The strange and the familiar may appear to be juxtaposed as we look at a photograph; if we study the picture intently, we may begin to see a familiar face differently. Captured on film, with a fleeting expression frozen upon their face, those who are close to us can begin to look quite unfamiliar, quite 'unlike themselves'. It would seem to be that this phenomenon has to do with the practice of repeatedly looking at a photograph of someone, in a way that we do not do with the 'real' person.

Staring at someone is not considered socially acceptable, so we rarely have the chance to fix our eyes on another person for longer than a few seconds. The photograph offers us this opportunity to stare for as long as we choose. Ample use may be made of this facility in therapy.

When the person is in our company, we generally look at the face. There are parts of the body that we are not 'allowed' to peruse at length in everyday social interaction. Each photograph offers us the prospect of gazing at leisure – at any part of the person at all. Perhaps it invites us to become voyeuristic.

The unusual experience that photographic gazing affords us produces its own phenomena. The resulting images can become quite bizarre in our minds, with certain features of the person becoming very noticeable and over-exaggerated. Having been focused on in this way, the people in the picture can begin to lose their identity in our eyes, become mere images, or collections of shapes, colours and textures.

The feelings engendered by this experience are perhaps comparable to those that we encounter when we endlessly repeat the same word, over and over again. It sometimes starts to sound strange and unfamiliar, so that we experiment with it, turn it round, maybe chant it repeatedly, give it a fresh rhythm, understand it anew, hear it differently.

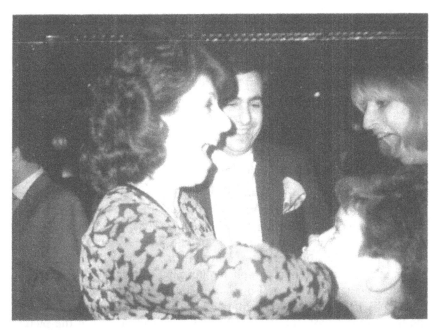

Photograph 5

A different way of telling . . .

Photography has a way of 'telling' that is immediate and straightforward. However, at the same time, it is also a circuitous and indirect method of communication.

To illustrate this duality, look at Photograph 5. Here there is sound, yet no sound, a definite story, yet none is told. We can make a good guess at what might be happening, from the facial expressions, gestures and body positions of the subjects. The child on the right has obviously said something shocking or embarrassing. The woman on the left covers up his mouth, and is herself exclaiming 'loudly'. She is also obviously amused. She looks at the woman on the right, who laughs out 'loud', in response. Behind, the man looks at the child with an expression of amused indulgence. The child himself has smiling, mischievous eyes.

This is a very 'noisy' picture, yet we cannot hear a sound. For photographs speak to us – and they are silent in the talking. They may shout out at us – but they do so mutely. They may talk to us, tell us a story, but without words.

Whilst we can gather a good deal of the story from this expressive picture, we can only do so in a general way. We cannot know exactly what has happened, despite the clarity of the images. For this, we need the narrative of someone who was present at the time. As I am the woman on the left of the picture, I hope I can be relied upon to give an accurate story.

This photograph was taken at a wedding, and I had been dancing with the man in the background, the husband of the woman to the right of the picture. As she approached, after the dance had finished, my son, then aged 9, addressing himself to her husband and me, asked in a clear, loud voice: 'Are you two having an affair?'

Perhaps now the picture's meaning falls into place . . .

Time paradoxes and the photograph: the instant and the eternal

I might have entitled the picture 'An embarrassing moment'. For the photographer has fortuitously captured the exact moment – seconds later and it would have been lost forever. The expressions would have changed, and the significance of the photograph would have disappeared. For that second, the world stopped, and the instant was preserved for posterity.

The subjects in the photograph remain unchanged, unaffected by the relentless march of time. As I make this statement, however, I am aware that, in itself, it is is obviously paradoxical. For the world did not stop, the moment did pass and it has gone forever. The people in the picture have grown older, the child has lost his youthful, mischievous innocence, the child is no longer a child. The instant and the eternal are both embodied in a photograph, confounding and perplexing us.

The photograph represents a fixed moment, yet it is also part of a continuous time-stream. It is timeless, in that it captures an image forever, whilst simultaneously being dependent for its very existence on split-second timing, the capturing of a moment. Time is splintered by the camera into miniscule parts. These can exist alone, yet they also have a vital place in the vast span of time. Thus, each picture has validity in its own right, and also in a relational way, as part of a sequence, a process. Each tiny moment is a section in the whole of the cycle. Such photographic time paradoxes can be haunting and disturbing, yet they merit considerable thought and study. They can enable us to learn new truths about ourselves and the world, putting the past into storage, to be reviewed and perhaps reframed in the present.

The photograph is a perpetual reminder of something transient; an elusive moment in an impermanent life that is recorded for posterity. It remains the same; but it does not. For, in itself it may age, become crumpled and cracked, torn and faded; thus it emphasises the progression of time by its own physical condition. The photograph gives meaning to life by verifying that the people depicted in it existed; simultaneously it reveals that they are merely shadows, perhaps long gone, almost meaning-less in the scheme of things. It can confirm the hollowness of one's transient and fragile existence, so that, like Shakespeare's Macbeth, we feel that 'Life's but a walking shadow, a poor player that struts and frets his hour upon the stage and then is heard no more' (5.V.ii.).

As we face the moment in our photograph, we are made aware of the limits of our mortality, because we know that the picture represents the snatching of a single instant out of eternity, an endlessness in which we have no part. In plucking out a moment of time from infinity, the camera highlights the measureless difference between the two.

Seeing yesterday today

As we have seen in Chapter 1, photographs can simultaneously reflect past, present and future in a weird kind of time-warp. We can even observe what the world was like long before our birth. We can see yesterday today. Our manner of talking about photographs and our way of using them reflect these time paradoxes; thus we are are often compelled to speak in the contradictory terms connected with the photographic medium.

Frequently, when newspapers are describing an event in the recent past, they illustrate this verbal confusion, precipitated by the photographic time paradox. Past and present are thoroughly mixed up, creating grammatical and semantic nonsense. We have become so used to this confusion in terms of the camera, that we hardly notice the contradictions. It seems, therefore, perfectly natural to display photographs with such captions as:

Supply Officer David Gatenby on the *Sir Galahad* and his girlfriend Miss Andrea Rudkin wave farewell yesterday.

(*Daily Telegraph*, 9 October 1990)

Ken Dodd, with plastic carrier bag, leaves home to give evidence at Liverpool crown court yesterday.

(*Daily Telegraph*, 7 July 1989)

It is natural, that is, until we really give the matter some thought . . . what was and what is become muddled through a visual presentation that shows a past event 'happening' in the now.

Photographs also reveal and compare what was, and what was not; they highlight the contrast between what occurred in a person's life and what was missing. One may become painfully aware of the lack of certain photographs; frequently these are pictures reflecting wished-for experiences. Paradoxically, the photographs that are present in an album can accentuate the absence of other pictures that were never taken.

New truths for old: fragmentation and reconstruction

Imagine: a pile of photographs falls to the floor. They lie scattered, moments of disconnected time. Photography fragments and reduces reality into a mass of parts that often appear to bear scant relation to the whole. It can also be a potent medium for reconstruction, reintegration and reclamation.

The photograph, whilst fracturing the flow of time, paradoxically can also contribute towards the restoration of an ordered progression, a linear whole. Photographs are inevitably selective and reductionist in that it is impossible to photograph everything, and there are many factors, like the photographer's own attitude to his or her subject, that will influence the finished result. Yet by gathering several photographs together, grouping them, gazing at the result, pondering on the new angles thus produced, one can gain a new and informative view of, for example, a lost past.

Exposure to many different photographs of the same subject, taken from various angles and viewpoints, seems to counteract the reductionist aspect and enable reconstruction.

Just as there are no two faces or fingerprints the same, so there are no photographs, even of the same person or scene, that exactly resemble each other. Collections of similar photographs can therefore be used to discover more of the whole story.

Historically, this method can be used to piece together destroyed towns or villages; it has been used to reconstruct the Warsaw Ghetto. At Yad Vashem, the Holocaust Memorial Centre in Jerusalem, the many different photographs of the Warsaw Ghetto have been used to build up a composite impression of both the people and the setting. Minute details are observed and linked on various photographs; landmarks, street names and shop signs give valuable clues and help the pictures to be fitted together mentally to build up a more complete scenario.

There are many diaries from this Ghetto in existence, and these, together with testimonies from the survivors, make the task less difficult. The diaries show, for example, that in the Ghetto an address was an intrinsic part of a person's identity and individuality. Each time a name was mentioned, an address automatically followed. Implicitly, therefore, as the buildings and houses are reassembled and related to each other the Ghetto becomes in some measure peopled and revivified.

From this intense photographic study, something of the Ghetto inhabitants' lives and routines has been reclaimed, rescued from oblivion. For example, the same Jewish Ghetto policeman can be seen in several pictures and it is possible from these appearances to chart much of this man's daily routine. Through this kind of work, we can learn more about history and about the social aspects of a lost people. Such an approach also has a psychologically restorative function. This kind of photographic reconstruction has echoes in the therapeutic situation, where the patient retrieves and reclaims his/her past. It will be seen later in this book how, using childhood pictures, the patient works towards rebuilding a split self, transforming and integrating the fragmented parts. Through understanding how the shattered pieces interrelate, one can construct a more meaningful whole. So it is in therapy. So it is in history.

The great paradox of life and death

What of the monumental themes of life and death, which create a multitude of eternal paradoxes to perplex us all? They are indeed inextricably linked through the photograph, mirroring the complexities inherent in the connection. The puzzle is reflected in the paradoxical story by Ibn Zabara: 'A man who lost his brother was asked, "What was the cause of his death?" and replied, "Life"' (Rosten 1977: 300).

Photographs preserve images of those we have lost, keeping them alive in our memory, perpetually available for constant and comforting scrutiny. Yet they simultaneously confront us with the fact of such loss, confirming how time has passed and how the loved one no longer exists. Whilst the picture of a lost relative may afford us some reassurance and company, it also underlines the yawning chasm between life and death. The comfort also encloses the pain. For the lost one is here, and not here.

In the poem 'Album', there is an awareness of the photographic phenomena of space and time. Puzzled by its complexity, the poet stares at the picture of himself and his family and says: 'I am here, I am there.' Both are true. Yet the photographic truth is paradoxical. He is there, in the photograph, but he cannot be there, because he is here, looking at it.

The photographic act can 'cause' both life and death. It can be, in its own peculiar way, death-dealing, for it freezes its subjects into eternity for looking into its lens. Movement is totally suspended and fixed forever. Perhaps this has overtones of the biblical story of Lot's wife, turned into a pillar of salt as a punishment for looking back to Sodom and Gomorrah.

Yet the same photograph can 'miraculously' bring to life a lost moment, or a deceased person; it can help to awaken the past, revivify the dead. This aspect of the photograph makes it a most useful adjunct to therapies concerned with loss and bereavement. It will be seen in Chapter 7 how photographs may render the lost person available, so that patients may once again be in touch with feelings and fantasies about people who are far away, or dead. Yet, in reality these people are inaccessible, out of touch; closeness and proximity in a physical way are a figment of the imagination. The photograph is thus both satisfying and unsatisfying, rewarding and frustrating, useful and useless.

Science and magic

The poem at the beginning of this chapter opens with the lines:

My father is dead.
I who am look at him
Who is not . . .

How can we look at someone who is not? Photography, through a kind of illusive magic, permits us to look upon someone who is alive, when he is in fact dead.

As we saw in Chapter 1, there is a certain magic about the camera for many people. From start to finish, the photographic process is one that can enchant children and adults alike. It is fascinating to capture a moment, to rescue it from invisibility. There is also magic in the taking, the developing and in the subsequent holding onto the photograph as a kind of good-luck charm.

Photographs 'conjure up' for us all sorts of images, sensations and experiences, invoking spirits of the past. In our albums, our younger selves, and the people with whom we have grown up, emerge from the pages like apparitions. Often they surprise us with their presence, as they materialise unexpectedly, mysterious phantoms belonging to a time past – 'Look! Suddenly/the young tool in their hands/for hurting one another.' The album lets us leaf through our life, become an onlooker, a reader of our own personal history book, in an almost surrealistic fashion.

At the same time, there is absolutely *nothing* magical or mysterious about the photograph at all. It is the product of a clear technical process, totally explainable in scientific terms.

Wounding and healing

The poem 'Album' at the beginning of this chapter reflects another contradictory aspect of the photograph. The lines 'there is no wound/time gives that is not bandaged by time' are highly relevant; the photograph has the potential to wound as well as to heal. It can be used in a negative or positive way. This will be seen most vividly in Chapter 6. Photographs of disturbing events in people's lives, or those evoking distressing memories can be used by some to heal and to work through trauma, whereas to others they are too painful and invasive to be in any way therapeutic. Therapists need to be acutely aware of this paradox in assessing patients for photo-therapy.

The photographer's dilemma

In relation to Holocaust photographs, there persists a somewhat disturbing photographic paradox in terms of aesthetics. A photographer will naturally want results to be artistically pleasing. This is all very well if the subject is a pleasant garden, a beautiful child, a majestic seascape. But what if the camera is being used to record human misery, degradation and suffering?

This dilemma was painfully experienced by George Rodger, who was the first to photograph Belsen concentration camp soon after it was liberated in 1945. He reflects:

I didn't know until then – despite over five years of war – what effect the war had on me personally . . . when I discovered that I could look at the horrors of Belsen – the 4000 dead and starving lying around – and think only of a nice photographic composition, I knew something had happened to me, and it had to stop.

(Rodger 1987: 7)

It would appear that, whilst Rodger's guilt and discomfort are understandable, to some extent his feelings are connected with an inescapable and unavoidable photographic paradox.

Perhaps achieving an aesthetic result may also be a defensive strategy on the part of the photographer, a way of avoiding the full impact of the horrors before him.

Ordinariness and beauty

Even without conscious effort on the part of the photographer to arrange an aesthetically pleasing picture, a kind of beauty is to be found in the most disturbing of subjects.

Connected with this is the fact that the camera invariably gives people or objects some kind of distinctive meaning, relevance and status (Sontag 1987: 28). It brings out the inherent qualities in the miserable, the poor and the oppressed, so that they become dramatically interesting. This is a paradoxical aspect of photographs that has echoes in therapeutic work. If one focuses on the most depressed, sad and colourless patient, looking beneath the superficial and defensive exterior, there is most often some spark of life, some unique, individual aspect that defines that person.

At the other end of the spectrum, photographs often present us with a perfect or ideal image, which invites further scrutiny and exploration. The camera can hide imperfections and conceal flaws that we know to be there.

Knowing

Many contradictions and paradoxes reside within the issue of knowing in relation to photographs. The photographer Diane Arbus has observed: 'A photograph is a secret about a secret. The more it tells, the less you know' (quoted in Sontag 1987: 111). This illusory quality contrasts with the apparently obvious immediacy of the snapshot. There is revelation and also concealment.

The photograph can be an aid to memory, and at the same time it can disconcertingly highlight the fact that there are memories that we cannot consciously recall. This is graphically illustrated by the writer Sylvia Fraser in her book *My Father's House*, about her own history of sexual abuse. Calling her chapter 'Mirror, Mirror', she describes her feelings on looking at some early photographs: 'A tinted photograph of my sister and of me hangs on the bedroom door of my Toronto duplex. I put it there soon after I remembered my father had sexually abused me.'

She then describes the photographs in some detail and continues:

A photograph album repeats these images – always the discomfited older child is behind the younger, who grins for the camera, her clothes exhibiting what might be called seductive details. . . . From time to time, I find myself staring into that cherubic face in the photograph. 'Tell me, little girl, what do you still know that I don't know?'

(Fraser 1989: 225)

The photograph thus helps us to know with its clarity and ability to preserve and expose the past, yet it also hinders us from knowing by its silence and ambiguity. The known and the unknown are embodied in a single picture; we are helped to understand, and we are also mystified. The photograph is therefore both reliable and disappointing, comforting and disturbing.

It is disconcerting to be faced in a picture with material that is unavailable to the conscious mind; however, another paradox arises when previously unconscious memories are triggered by the photograph: we then come to know what, at some level, we have known all along.

Words from an old Zen story put this concept succinctly: 'Thank you Master for teaching me nothing' (Brandon 1976: 24). Many times, as we look into our photographs, we see – or we do not see – what we know to be true. Our subsequent learning, therefore, is in actuality a reawakening of awareness, repressed and hidden in our unconscious until prompted by the visual cue.

The following Talmudic extract also describes a similar way of looking at the concept of learning:

Before a child is born, a light is held
behind its head with which it can see
from one end of the world to the other,
and they teach it the whole of the Torah.
But at the moment of birth an angel
touches it on the lips, and it forgets all.
So all of life is spent remembering
what we once knew.

(from Blue 1985: 40)

PARADOXES IN THERAPY AND THEIR PHOTOGRAPHIC REFLECTIONS

Several of the paradoxes related to the photograph directly reflect the ambivalent issues that are the stuff of therapy, and they also mirror aspects of the therapy itself. These links and connections are considered here.

Paradoxical images: the incomplete self

Patients often enter therapy because, consciously or unconsciously, they are beset by inner ambivalent and conflicting feelings that may be suppressed and hidden from awareness. Such feelings lie, unacknowledged, rumbling beneath other facets of the personality which, whilst being neither false nor unreal, are simply less difficult to express. They are just a part of the story, not the whole of it. There develops a one-sided self which conceals behaviour, fantasies and feelings that conflict and jar against the socially acceptable self-image.

The paradox of the one-sided self is that it conceals and contains its opposite. So, the most passive and polite patient in therapy, who is most anxious to please the therapist, may be suppressing rage and violence beneath the surface. On further exploration, this over-anxiety to please is found to conceal just the opposite kind of feelings – a real anger and hatred towards the therapist and all that she represents for the patient.

This psychological mechanism is called 'reaction formation'; long years of repressing 'unacceptable' feelings have resulted in a move to the other extreme, in an attempt to camouflage the inadmissible. Such intolerable feelings may unconsciously be very threatening, for they may have been condemned and forbidden by years of parental admonition, threats of punishment, withdrawal of love and outright rejection.

Children are soon forced to deny such feelings (most often these are rage, anger, sadness, yearning) and develop a one-sided way of being that becomes the norm and is carried into adult life. They 'forget' they ever had another self. Unconsciously, they know that such feelings must not be discovered, paradoxically even by themselves. So strong is the fear, that the feelings become terrifying inner monsters, ever growing in the face of attempts to bridle and restrain them.

When people enter therapy with such incomplete selves, it is difficult to gain any kind of rounded image of them as people. From birth, they may not have felt *seen*; somehow they did not have a true enough reflection of themselves mirrored back to them in early life.

The ensuing cover-up may be efficient, but it can feel questionable in some way to the therapist; she will be alerted in any case by the extreme nature of the masking behaviour. This partial presentation of self in therapy is not generally able to disguise all the inner conflicts and contradictions; there will inevitably be whispers from the un-conscious about them, subtle communications of their existence. The unconscious mind will reveal its messages covertly, perhaps through almost imperceptible signs. These may take the form of a mismatch between words and expressions, or a thought-less gesture that signifies hidden and conflicting feelings and motivations, despite overt verbal messages to the contrary.

Not quite as simple as its seems . . .

Our photographs can confront us with the existence of such confusing, disturbing clashes and inconsistencies that beset us internally and externally in our daily lives. If we are able to look beneath the surface, we can use the photograph in therapy to help us focus and concentrate on any incongruities, either in what we perceive in the picture, or in the feelings we have about it. Such discrepancies may indicate that there is more to the picture than meets the eye, and may help us to identify unconscious conflicts.

The simplicity of a snapshot belies its intricacy. Easily taken, lightly perused, its clear images may appear facile, uncomplicated, even shallow. Yet, once a personally relevant photograph is studied with a more perceptive attitude, it becomes something less obvious and more enigmatic. Perhaps it may develop into an object of profound significance.

The photograph is double-sided, two-faced. The ability to see beyond the sur-face is dependent on the viewer's capacity to think psychologically and their skill in looking beneath the veneer of the first impression. Only then will the paradoxical nature of what is seen emerge and become apparent. Otherwise the photograph, capable of revealing so much, will hide its secrets. This is a classic example of the paradoxical statement 'I can't see for looking.'

Many people have boxes of family and personal photographs that contain clues about their history, relationship patterns and generational problems. Unless they are viewed with a perceptive eye, they will remain like puzzle drawings that conceal hidden shapes, available to be seen only after concentrated perusal. Thus, photographs secrete their mysteries beneath a façade of manifest images. Beyond the visible may lurk invisible feelings, thoughts and attitudes that may give the lie to the apparently cheerful and happy faces.

The photograph may camouflage the truth, masking the considerable energy used in the struggle to exercise control over the unconscious. For this threatens to emerge unbounded and unchecked, endangering a fragile equilibrium and conflicting with a meticulously designed, yet fragmentary, self-image. There is often a flatness in this image, producing a lack of vigour and a dullness in people who deny all 'negatives' in themselves. This superficial image is also what faces us when we give a photograph no more than a cursory glance. There is a blandness, an insipid quality to the two-dimensional image if we see only its surface.

However, whilst the photograph may appear flat and insubstantial, if our minds are receptive, we can see into it in a way that shows its depth and essence. Beyond the profusion of smiles and the multitude of 'acceptable' selves, are their contradictory opposites. They remain to be discovered if only we dare face their direct reflections inside us. If we can bear to confront, explore and examine them, then perhaps we can come to terms with them, with less denial, suppression or division. It will be seen in Chapters 3 and 4 that photographs, used therapeutically, can assist in the discovery of the inner self, helping one to see the whole person beneath the one-sided appearance.

Just as, in therapy, we explore behaviour on a reality, surface level, and on a deeper, unconscious level, so we need to explore the photograph in this dual way. The two levels may appear inconsistent. In the photograph, this masking behaviour may also be apparent; people frequently cover up painful feelings with smiles, and sometimes they are not too successful (see Photograph 9).

It must be reiterated here that emotional health is in part dependent upon an acceptance of the fact that ambiguities and contradictions exist, both internally and externally. If, for example, we can accept that it is possible to experience both love and hate towards one and the same person, then we will come to accept the contradictory nature of our emotions. These opposites within us can then have some kind of unified existence. Like major and minor musical keys, which together create a melodious symphony, opposing aspects within the personality can construct a harmonious whole, by means of the discord.

The paradox in the pose

Photographs can represent spontaneously snatched moments in a person's life, capturing subjects unaware, or when relaxing. They can also be posed and measured, structured and directed.

The photographic pose may be seen as reflecting aspects of the presentation of the one-sided self in therapy. A pose is inevitably a contradiction; it is about wanting to appear to be something one is not; to create an image that fits in with the subject's wishes – or maybe those of the photographer. When one is photographed, there is usually a desire to look one's 'best'.

Perhaps one might also want to appear cheerful when sad, or part of a happy family group when there is trauma – to deny reality through the camera. There are, however, many tell-tale signs, straight from the unconscious, that give away the secrets that the pose partially obscures (see Photograph 13 and accompanying narrative).

It is helpful for the therapist to be able to detect and recognise such unconscious or hidden signs in a photograph: they are so often pointers to important themes in relationships that may need further examination. Once spotted, these oblique signals often contrast sharply with the overall tone of the photograph. Thus, the general impression of the photograph becomes less uniform, more ambiguous. Symptoms of a deeper disharmony emerge. These signs may appear irritating or nonsensical, and it may be tempting to disregard or dismiss them impatiently.

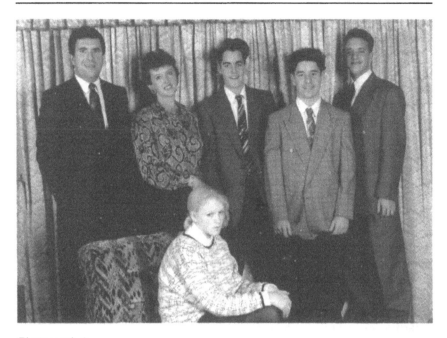

Photograph 6
Posed by models

At other times, there may be discovered more obvious contrasts and discrepancies in a photograph that may perhaps be seen as a kind of message.

This is illustrated in the case of Diana, who brought to therapy a photograph of herself with her family as a teenager, taken on the occasion of her brother's birthday. The whole family appeared happy and they were all smiling – except Diana (Photograph 6). She looked sullen and miserable. The intention of the photographer had obviously been to take a 'good' photograph, a happy snap for the album. For Diana, the picture – and many others like it – expressed her unhappy rebellion and discomfort within a family that felt to her alien and rejecting. Even though it was not *her* birthday, she felt she was the focus of the picture, in a kind of negative way, making her appear the odd one out. This graphically symbolised her feelings in her family, where she constantly felt that she was singled out as different from the others. In therapy, we were able to focus on these feelings through the photograph – obviously with a very different understanding of it from the actual photographer.

However incidental they may appear, such small details of behaviour are intended to be a communication. In a similar way, many patients who come into therapy display all kinds of behaviour that may at first glance appear bizarre, eccentric, peculiar or downright infuriating. If one explores and works with the behaviour, rather than immediately attempting to eliminate it, there will emerge clues to the real feelings beneath. So often the 'strange' behaviour is a kind of paradoxical way of asking for help.

It may be that attempts to reach others have become distorted by painful past experience; perhaps the patient has not felt heard or has had to control real expressions of need. However, these confused efforts at communicating inner feelings often produce the opposite reactions to those desired and are met with impatience and rejection. Diana was at some level communicating her anger, need and distress through her sad face – yet she received only more criticism from her family for 'bad' behaviour after the photograph was developed. Her general attitude was regarded as incomprehensible by many who came across her – why be so 'difficult' in such an apparently happy family?

Direction and no direction

The photograph can give us direction in some ways, and not in others. The edges of the picture limit it in terms of space; an outer frame prevents us from moving outside the picture on a physical level, directing our attention within. In addition, through its structure and composition, the photograph leads the eye from shape to shape. This is especially true of professionally taken photographs, where considerable attention is given to composition and form. On the other hand, there is no direction; we are free to explore the images in any sequence we choose: 'A picture has no particular direction and is thus extra-temporal in that it does not insist on being "read" in any order' (Holmes 1985: 251).

The photograph lingers and remains constant for our perusal, waiting for us to notice it, to read deeper if we will, to roam psychically beyond its physical borders. But it issues no guidance. It is ready to be what we wish, to be interpreted in any way we choose, or to be left, coded and cryptic, undeciphered.

The same paradox is true of therapy. There is form and structure, and there is not; within a secure framework of therapeutic boundaries, patient and therapist are free to explore and wander, to linger and wait without constraint. There is no overt map or plan in terms of the way material from the patient's unconscious will be used. The patient is free to read and interpret this material according to choice – in any order – within the framework of the therapy hour.

There is also the freedom to set aside or leave unexplored any difficult symbols or issues which may emerge, if the patient feels unready – or unwilling – to confront them. They may be left at the level of the symbolic, not brought into consciousness and given only cursory regard. Perhaps they will be 'filed away', to be looked at again at a more appropriate time.

The paradox of the transference and its reflections in the photograph

The photograph's duality is reflected in so many areas of our experience; it can represent reality and fantasy, conscious and unconscious, inner and outer, past and present, child and adult. If we are able to utilise it therapeutically, then the duality in a photograph can help us to bring about real change. The firm knowledge that in reality it is safe and familiar, having no substantial power to harm us, helps us to venture into the less certain level of the unconscious, the insecure world of childhood fears and feelings.

The frame of the photograph is firmly there to remind us that this is an 'as if' situation (Milner 1977: 131); it may be compared to the edges of the screen in a film, which limits the borders of the action and tells us that we are witnessing a representation of life, not life itself. The photograph frames and contains the past in the present, so that we can enter the boundless realms of yesteryear. Thus we are able to revisit and confront people who figured large in our lives, perhaps remembering and re-experiencing a whole range of emotions and exploring fears and fantasies.

We may encounter in a photograph the outer representation of internalised figures and feelings from the past, deeply buried within our psyche. These may feel very real and threatening, even though they are now just memories. It may be that in time, having faced these, we may come to 'reframe' the past, seeing it in a new light. We may discover a new way of being, having remembered, re-experienced and taken leave of the old.

The paradoxes inherent in this therapeutic use of the photograph are reflected in the transference within the therapy situation. The therapist may come to represent, metaphorically, a figure from the past and the patient will re-experience early feelings towards her. The paradox is contained in the metaphor – the patient feels as if the therapist were really a childhood figure. If, for example, there has been an experience of abandonment by mother in childhood, there is likely to be fear of this from the therapist, experiencing her, symbolically, as the parent who will again let the patient down.

Simultaneously, the patient knows that the therapist is a professional in the here-and-now, and is *not* that parent, which creates a feeling of safety. In addition, therapeutic boundaries function to frame and make safe the patient's experience. It is important that there is in the therapy some similarity to a past relationship in the patient's mind to enable feelings and fantasies to emerge. There must, however, be enough difference to be bearable; too complete a resemblance to the past would recreate an intolerable situation for the patient.

There is thus a valuable paradox in the therapist's role for the patient, which will enable a recreation of past emotional scenarios. The patient will most often anticipate similar reactions from the therapist to the ones experienced in the past, confirming a negative self-image. Whilst the patient may not consciously remember significant aspects of past relationships, the manner of relating to the therapist will be significant in gaining an understanding of past experiences. Transference is a way of unconsciously remembering. The patient will inevitably repeat past relationship patterns in therapy, manifesting the manner of relating which has been familiar in the past. Only through sensitive interpretation of the transference, will such patterns be brought to consciousness.

The patient who, for example, has felt constantly put down and criticised in childhood, will anticipate this attitude from the therapist. For a long while, such a person cannot dare to believe that the reaction from the therapist will be any different from the negativity he or she has known. The therapist, in remaining an accepting and non-judgemental figure for the patient, facilitates a different experience in therapy this time, thus breaking the vicious circle of negativity in which the patient has been trapped.

Such vicious circles can be vividly reflected through photographs; generations in a family can be condemned by lack of awareness into compulsively and remorselessly repeating the same destructive relationship patterns. As the therapist helps the patient to recognise and identify these hitherto unconscious ways of being, such photographs can aid awareness and recognition of patterns of behaviour. They can also help to correct negative personal and family myths and fantasies that have persisted over time.

Sarah continually expected me to see her as a 'bad, ugly girl' and brought me several childhood photographs to 'prove' this. In the transference, she saw me as the mother who was competitive with her, and envious of her, and who would always compare her unfavourably with others. At one level, she knew that this was untrue, and remained in therapy because of this knowledge and the hope that for once she might have a different experience. She observed closely my reaction to her pictures, looking for signs of rejection, testing me, almost willing me to rebuff her. She found it hard to believe that I was not grimacing at the images. I saw nothing to reject. She was the one who now labelled herself in a deprecating way.

Slowly, she risked trusting that I would not react as she had expected and she produced yet more pictures, and actually started to see for herself the sad, isolated, attractive little girl beneath the 'bad' label. The paradoxical nature of the transference relationship had enabled Sarah to express her fears and fantasies with me, in an atmosphere that felt dangerous (past, fantasy, inner world) and also safe (present, reality, outer world). The duality of the photographs had meant that unsafe, past feelings and fantasies could be expressed within the security of the knowledge that there was a frame of safety around them, a secure enough therapeutic environment.

Safety and danger are thus inherent in both the transference and the photograph, and this produces a kind of therapeutic tension. This tension is a necessary factor in achieving creative change, because the patient needs enough safety to be able to open up and enough confrontation to stimulate new ways of seeing. It is important that each balances the other out, so that the pain may be felt and enclosed within the safety – and that the atmosphere of the session is neither too comfortable nor too threatening. When photographs are brought to therapy, their paradoxical aspects mirror that of the transference, as they confirm, parallel and echo the dual nature of so many facets of the patient's experience.

SPOTTING THE PHOTOGRAPHIC PARADOX: SEEING CREATIVELY

In order to sharpen her perceptions and develop the ability to detect such paradoxes, the therapist needs to foster within herself a different way of seeing. This will involve a creative and therapeutic kind of mind-stretching, so that she becomes psychologically agile and flexible enough to detect photographic paradoxes. Only then will she be able to help patients recognise and accept the reflections of these visual paradoxes inside themselves.

How can this be achieved? In developing an innovative attitude as we look at the world around us, we can become increasingly inventive in the mental exercises that we set ourselves in relation to our surroundings. It is important to strive to expand and extend our awareness, exploring our world with an increasingly adaptable attitude.

This will entail a breaking of habitual ways of seeing and perceiving the world. These may feel safe enough, but are ultimately restrictive. It is all too easy to become cushioned by convention into a comfortable existence, yet one that is stultifying to creativity.

Gestalt therapy may provide us with a way to start extricating ourselves from the rut of routine and habit. By developing the skill of seeing things in reverse, the mind becomes freer and less rigid in its functioning:

> Consider some everyday life-situations, objects or activities as if they were *precisely the opposite* of what you customarily take them to be. Imagine yourself in a situation the reverse of your own, where you have inclinations and wishes exactly contrary to your usual ones. Observe objects, images and thoughts as if their function or meaning were the antithesis of what you habitually take them to be. Furthermore, confronting them thus, hold in abeyance your standard evaluations of good and bad, desirable or repugnant, sensible or silly, possible or impossible. Be satisfied to stand between them – at the zero-point, interested in both sides of the opposition but not siding with either.
>
> (Perls *et al.* 1951: 45 6)

A way of beginning may be to attempt to reverse statements you yourself have made, discovering some opposites there. Instead of saying 'Mary doesn't like me', try 'I don't like Mary', and see how it feels. It may also contain a truth that may surprise you.

Pushing further, maybe into the realms of the surreal, begin mentally turning things on their heads. Design an upside-down, topsy-turvy world, where trees have branches that spread and push deep into the earth, and roots that stretch themselves upwards to the sky. Allow yourself to be ridiculous and uninhibited in your experimenting.

Take a look at the people around you – your parents, children, your partner or spouse. Imagine them doing things they do not usually do, saying the unexpected. Marital therapists work on the principle that we express for our spouse the feelings and behaviours that he or she may find difficult, and vice versa. If your spouse is shy or retiring, picture him or her as the opposite kind of person. In your mind let your partner be loud, excitable, bombastic. If you have married an 'angry' person, imagine the other to be calm and cool, and put yourself in the angry role. Give him/her a break from carrying a 'double dose' of one particular kind of behaviour.

Maybe you will discover deep truths about yourself and your partner, coming face to face with hitherto repressed feelings. In Chapter 6, we will explore further ways in which to develop the mind, and explore the self-image with a view to encouraging creativity.

Double thinking, double vision

When we are confronted with a paradox in a photograph, it is important to take note of the dissonance, for it may inform us in some way. In order to stay with the contradictions, we need to develop a facility for a kind of double thinking, viewing the paradox as a potential source of insight.

It is important for therapists using photographs to go outside their usual frame of reference, expand awareness, using paradoxical concepts in a therapeutic way. This attitude will challenge set practices, provide a jolt to those who have fixed attitudes, allowing a new way of seeing. Family therapists have long since discovered the healing power of the paradox, working with the symptom, rather than trying to erase it.

Perhaps, unwittingly, we may have used this method already with our children. Parents with frayed nerves, having urged their children to go to bed several times and to no avail, may often end up saying 'OK, stay up all night. That's quite alright by us.' This often does the trick quicker than all the 'logical' requests.

Re-editing and reframing

Often, as children, 'realities' have been constructed for us, and we begin to see ourselves through the eyes of others. Like Sarah, the 'bad, ugly child' described above, we may absorb unhealthy family mythology, which tends, if it is excessive, to blunt our perceptions. We may have been pressed into a mould, fashioned and shaped according to the will of others. The resulting image is an amalgam of outside influences, a composite blend of familial, cultural and social constructions and manipulations. If we have rebelled against these constructions, donning the mantles of opposition emotionally and physically, our true selves still remain hidden beneath a mask of defiance.

Photographs can be used to re-edit the past and challenge the myths and legends that have been cultivated about us and with which we have colluded during the period of growing up. Their exploration gives us the chance to shift the fixed image, to see the other side of the picture and, paradoxically, to alter what we perceive without altering it.

Through the medium of reframing, we can help others to come to terms with unmanageable or intolerable dilemmas. In their book *Change*, Watzlawick *et al.* explain the concept:

> To reframe, then, means to change the conceptual and/or emotional setting or viewpoint in relation to which a situation is experienced and to place it in another frame which fits the 'facts' of the same concrete situation equally well or even better, and thereby changes its entire meaning. The mechanism involved here is not immediately obvious, especially if we bear in mind that there is change while the situation itself may remain quite unchanged and, indeed, even unchangeable. What turns out to be changed as a result of reframing is the meaning attributed to the situation, and therefore its consequences, but not its concrete facts – or, as the philosopher Epictetus expressed it as early as the first century A.D., 'It is not the things themselves which trouble us, but the opinions that we have about these things.'
>
> (Watzlawick *et al.* 1974: 95)

The philosopher is revealing an ancient truth – he knows that the power for change and growth is within us. Reframing helps us to utilise this power, to adjust our ways of seeing, to create an innovative blend of old and new. Those who use this technique know that it enables an expansion of vision, an adjustment of the 'opinions' that have troubled us. They have an awareness that truth is multi-faceted and a firm belief in the healing potential of the paradox. They have identified paradox as an effective aid to understanding and change because it extends the boundaries of logic beyond received opinion.

Etymologically, the word is derived from the Greek 'para-', meaning 'beyond' and 'doxa', meaning 'opinion'. It involves the cultivation of an attitude that is contrary to the popular view of the world, a view that goes beyond 'common sense'. When this way of seeing is applied to the photograph, it becomes apparent that if we wish to discover the essential truths within, to see beyond the smile, we also have to reach 'beyond opinion'. To some extent, this means ridding oneself of the preconceptions and convictions that may have made us set in our ways.

An old Zen story illustrates this well:

'A Cup of Tea'

Nan-in, a Japanese master . . . received a university professor who came to inquire about Zen.

Nan-in served tea. He poured his visitor's cup full, and then kept on pouring.

The professor watched the overflow until he no longer could restrain himself. 'It is overfull. No more will go in!'

'Like this cup,' Nan-in said, 'you are full – of opinions and speculations. How can I show you Zen unless you first empty your cup?'

(Reps 1989: 19)

Photographs present us with graphic images about which we may have troubling opinions. Then we need to examine the opinions, rather than the images. These pictures, intense and distinct, serve to provoke in us a clutter of mixed reactions, a confusing scatter of responses, comprised largely of feelings, judgements, myths and memories. They are triggered by the photographic images in a way that makes them accessible to consciousness, available to be challenged and reframed until their effect recedes.

ONE FINAL PARADOX . . .

There remains one final paradox that must not escape our notice. This can be vividly, graphically illustrated by the photograph; it concerns the theme of sameness and difference and it reflects the therapeutic relationship.

However, the particular photograph that I am visualising to illustrate the paradox is one that can rarely, if ever, be taken.

I therefore ask the reader to imagine it from my description:

Two people are sitting, opposite each other, yet at an angle, the one slightly leaning towards the other. They are obviously involved in some meaningful conversation, for they appear connected, absorbed. From their synchronised expressions and gestures, it is apparent that there is an interplay of thought and feeling, a rapport that holds them in a quite intense mutual exchange.

Can you guess what is happening, who these people may be?

They are, in fact, therapist and patient; but who could tell, in the instant of this photograph, which is which?

Paradoxically, they look similar, yet the sameness also contains the disparity, the resemblance contradicts the dissimilarity. Thus the photo-graph emphasises the mutuality of the therapeutic endeavour, whilst hiding the secret of the different roles and identities. Whilst the therapist maintains an open and empathic attitude, working in a co-operative and reciprocal way, she does not discuss her personal life or problems with her patient. It is most important that this somewhat paradoxical, 'mutual but asymmetrical', relationship (Hobson 1985: 37) is maintained throughout therapy.

I have shown in this chapter how important is an understanding of the notion of paradox when considering the therapeutic use of photographs. With this firmly in mind, and with an awareness of the mass of paradoxes inherent in the whole of the therapeutic process, I shall now move to a specific exploration of the use of photographs in therapy.

Chapter 3

Using photographs in therapy
Some general principles

'Snapshot of Me as a Boy'

I'm lonely in the ashen field
as an abandoned shack is lonely
but doesn't know it.

It's the last honest age, a depression
of mild and pallid silence, years
before the lie of color.

You others who ran after time
hoping to reach the present
see what you've missed?

Not one single gray leaf fallen
not a single black rose
of the hedge blown.
(Leonard Nathan, *Holding Patterns*)

In this chapter, I shall give an overview of the various methods of photo-therapy, and then proceed to a detailed discussion of the use of photographs in psychoanalytic psychotherapy.

DIFFERENT APPROACHES TO PHOTO-THERAPY

The ways in which photographs are used therapeutically are contrasting and varied. A multiplicity of methods may be applied; it is important to differentiate between the various approaches. They will reflect the contrasting styles of different therapists, the many schools of therapy, and also the various ways in which patients themselves choose to use photographs. Whatever the therapist's approach, however, it is important that she must have had the kind of solid and thorough training that will enable her to cope with the patient's difficult experiences in therapy, often triggered by photographic exploration.

The making of the photographs by the patient

This can either be done in the session, where the process in itself is therapeutic, or outside the session, where the patient also learns in a different way about choices – in terms of subject, settings, attitudes, etc. There are considerable advantages to patients here: they have power and control in their own hands, in a way they may not have experienced previously, and this will inevitably aid in the enhancement of self-esteem.

In his book *Photographing the Self*, Ziller outlines the positive effects of such active photo-therapy:

> The auto-photographic approach to observation is reflexive. There is an inherent partnership between the scientist and the subject. By giving the camera to the subject, the subject is given control, just as the scientist/observer communicates control when he/she is in possession of the camera. Thus, the camera is a symbol of control, and giving the camera to the subject is a symbolic gesture of shared control.
>
> The subject's responses – photographs – also create a positively weighted relationship between scientist and subject. Photographs tend to generate positive associations. This response derives in part from the 'miracle'-like quality of photographs. Through photography we instantly become artists. Moreover, we are able to communicate vast amounts of information effortlessly. Similarly, the viewer of the photograph is presented with a response which tends to have positive associations. There is a positive response set inherent in the photographic process.
>
> (Ziller 1990: 36–7)

Through perceiving what patients choose to photograph, the therapist is helped to become acquainted with their self-image and their relationships in the external world and she may also gain a glimpse into their own inner world. People may bring photographs they have taken of significant others in their lives, yet these still reflect the patients' own view of the world, in the way they have chosen to take them. They may also have some help to take self-portraits (see Chapter 7), so that they can discover more about themselves through the photographs.

In addition, some patients are asked to bring photographs that others have taken of them, as a way of learning more about the self, and gaining feedback from others. Individually, or in groups, they can explore the medium of photographs in an innovative way, discovering a multitude of different methods and techniques.

Therapists who have the skills and equipment help people to take and develop their own photographs inside the therapy, or indeed as a therapy in itself. As an alternative, the polaroid camera enables the taking of instant pictures, making images immediately available for scrutiny and exploration. Such photographic acts of self-expression may quite often represent a first-time experience for the patients, giving them a sense of self-esteem, responsibility and importance as individuals. Having themselves photographed means that they become centre-stage, attracting much needed attention and focus. In some cases the therapist herself takes photographs of the patient – 'before and after' pictures that may show growth and change.

Some people are encouraged to take metaphorical, symbolic photographs (of scenes, objects) and they use these to express their innermost feelings and fantasies, to communicate their inner landscapes to the outside world. Perhaps they will make of them photographic collages, centred around particular themes.

Krauss (1980: 8) suggests the construction of a family album if none exists; this enables people to design the life they would have liked to have, perhaps using others to help them with the photographs. Photographs can be posed in the here-and-now, to fill gaps in past experience, and this gives patients some kind of reconstructive experience and power over the course of their life in the future. Krauss also suggests the making of photographs that express 'What I would like to happen in the future', which seems an appropriate exercise to do towards the end of therapy.

The use of video provides an additional experience; here is an opportunity for people to observe themselves and others; to watch the movement that a photograph denies them, to have sounds and words preserved, always with the facility to replay, re-hear and re-view. One can observe communications and interactions as they occur on film, so that they can be examined and understood. The video serves as a measure of change, a permanent record of how we have been, and how we are today.

Photographs as projectives

Some therapists prepare their own photographic collections, choosing a wide range of subjects. For example, there may be a photograph of a child, playing happily with a large dog. Or there may be a more abstract images of water, leaves or sky.

The patient will be asked to choose a picture that particularly appeals, or is meaningful. Then, the photograph will be used as a basis for fantasy and free association. This process will be facilitated by the therapist, who will note her patient's responses and reactions, encouraged by her appropriate interpretations and questions. Such images will inevitably stimulate different reactions in different people, according to personality and experience. These reactions will indicate much about ways of seeing the self and the world; this method of photo-therapy may also provide a way into deep personal issues.

The patient's ready-made photographs

Patients may bring along to the therapy their own albums of personally selected photographs, showing aspects of their life-history and that of their family. Mostly, these will have been taken by parents, relatives, friends or, perhaps, by people unknown to the patient; on the other hand, some may have been taken by patients themselves. They make a choice in terms of selection of such photographs for therapy and may manipulate the completed pictures, but they have had no active part in their creation.

Photographs such as this serve to record what the photographer perceived and experienced at a moment in time past. In therapy, however, feelings, fantasies and associations are projected onto the completed images, frequently years after the taking of the picture. Here the photographs are received and viewed in therapy by patient and therapist with attitudes that must inevitably differ substantially from the original photographers' approach to and understanding of their subjects.

Emphasis must also be given at this point to the primary differences involved in the using of such ready-made photographs which are brought to therapy, and the more active making of the image by the patient, which I have described above. As I stated in the Preface, my preference is for such ready-made images, using them as an adjunct to the process of psychoanalytic therapy.

THE USE OF PHOTOGRAPHS IN PSYCHOANALYTIC PSYCHOTHERAPY

Concepts and processes

An examination of some of the concepts and processes that are relevant to psychoanalytical psychotherapy, and where photographs can fit into these, may be helpful in illustrating the immense value of photographs in therapy.

Photographs and memory: reflections from the unconscious

Photographs fulfil many powerful functions in psychoanalytic psychotherapy; above all, they provide us with a unique way into the unconscious. Through their exploration, patients can begin to get in touch with feelings, behaviours and experiences that may have been traumatic in the past. Photographs are helpful in this because they stimulate all kinds of memories. Emotional experiences are awakened as the images confront our senses, revivifying forgotten feelings, sparking associations in the present out of the dying embers of our past.

Sometimes the memories are less than conscious; these may be termed 'feeling-memories'; they powerfully assail the whole body, in the form of physical sensations; they are strong feelings whose source may be forgotten in the conscious mind. At other times, wholly-felt memories burst into awareness, seemingly from nowhere, activated by a sudden glance at an old scene. Such experiences, so frequently prompted by the sight of photographs, can also occur when our other senses are stimulated, such as hearing, smell or taste.

Something of the intensity of such unexpected encounters with the past is conveyed by Marcel Proust who recalls his feelings when he tasted a madeleine dipped in tea:

> No sooner had the warm liquid mixed with the crumbs touched my palate than a shudder ran through me and I stopped, intent upon the extraordinary thing that was happening to me. An exquisite pleasure had invaded my senses, something isolated, detached, with no suggestion of its origin . . .
>
> Whence could it have come to me, this all-powerful joy? I sensed that it was connected with the taste of the tea and the cake, but that it infinitely transcended those savours, could not, indeed be of the same nature. Whence did it come? What did it mean? How could I seize and apprehend it? . . .
>
> I put down the cup and examine my own mind. It alone can discover the truth. But how? What an abyss of uncertainty, whenever the mind feels overtaken by itself; when it, the seeker is at the same time the dark region through which it must go seeking and where all its equipment will avail it nothing. Seek? More than that: create. It is face to face with something which does not yet exist, to which it alone can give reality and substance, which it alone can bring into the light of day . . .
>
> Undoubtedly what is thus palpitating in the depths of my being must be the image, the visual memory which, linked to that taste, is trying to follow it into my conscious mind. But its struggles are too far off, too confused and chaotic; scarcely can I perceive the neutral glow into which the elusive whirling medley of stirred-up colours is fused, and I cannot distinguish its form . . .
>
> (Proust 1981: 48–9)

The photograph provides us with the form and the visual memory that Proust recaptured after considerable effort. We attach meaning and feelings to the photographic presentation of our past and may thus experience the kind of intense sensations that Proust has described.

This may be seen in the reactions to photographs of a 40-year-old patient, Klaus, who brought many pictures of his family from Germany. He felt sad about not knowing most of his relatives because of the Second World War; his parents had divorced when he was very young and he lived with his mother. He felt intensely deprived of fatherly attention, and longed for physical contact with a paternal figure; there was a great emptiness, a gap in his life. Occasionally, however, he was taken to visit his maternal grandfather; he remembers, then, that he frequently needed to clamber onto Grandad's knee and thus get into touch with the only male figure in his life. As Klaus looks at the photographs of his grandfather, he has an overwhelming feeling of how it was to touch him, and most especially to smell the warm smell of him, and the tobacco that lingered in his memory. 'In an instant,' Klaus reflects, 'the feeling and the smell of Grandad were strongly evoked by the picture, as well as my own loneliness and neediness of him. I felt almost overcome by the power of it all.'

Out of these images and sensations, stimulated by the photographs, came memories and feelings that formed a significant part of the subsequent therapy, enabling Klaus to begin to understand the roots of his present day problems in relationships. A fuller description of Klaus's exploration of his family album will be found in Chapter 6.

Shadows of the past

Many reasons for present anxiety, depression and relationship problems are linked to disturbing childhood experiences from where emotional needs may have remained, unheard and unmet. These unresolved issues, carried into adulthood, create problems within the self and in relationships. Whilst it may be possible – and indeed sometimes necessary – to repress the memories and feelings associated with such experiences or to sublimate them through activity during early adulthood, they may eventually surface, in a form that varies according to the individual's personality.

In some cases, such feelings may be wholly or partially repressed, and may then express themselves through a psychiatric or physical illness.

For some people, seemingly from nowhere, 'forgotten' pain emerges; panicky, fearful feelings arise from long years of dormancy. They are caught unawares, for such conflicts have been relegated to the realms of the unconscious in a past that may now be barely remembered. Frantically, and erroneously, there may be a search for events in the present to explain what is happening. Full blame will be apportioned, perhaps to marriage or job, which may indeed have served to trigger such an upsurge of painful feelings.

If there is no awareness of the roots of these feelings in the past, the discomfort persists, lingering like a nameless curse. As a result of such haunting emotional turmoil, there is withdrawal in fear from potential closeness with others, lest the wounds are jarred, by even the slightest emotional knock. Unless the damage is investigated, explored at its source, it carries with it a life sentence of discontent and destructive behaviour.

Photographs can reveal these unconscious ways of being though visually highlighting repeated generational patterns. We shall see in subsequent chapters how they may thus be used by patients in therapy to try to liberate themselves from the traps of the past.

Patients may have some insight into the roots of their problems, or they may have little awareness in this area. It must be stressed that the purpose of therapy is to help unconscious feelings, wishes and motivations to become more conscious, in the hope that these can be worked through, once patients become mindful of just how much they are troubling their internal world.

If childhood feelings are repressed, this is precisely because they are so disturbing. Therapy aims to help unblock difficult feelings so that fuller exploration of past traumas is facilitated – within the context of the transference relationship. In order to work towards resolution and healing, it is important to be able to confront troubling issues and emotions in depth without avoiding them. Photographs help us in this confrontation, in stimulating disturbing memories.

Through the influence of the psychotherapeutic setting, the patient will inevitably re-experience early childhood feelings and behaviour in the relationship with the therapist which have previously been relegated to the unconsious. Powerful primitive feelings are aroused through this process, which is termed regression; one of the most important functions of psychotherapy is to enable such regression. Photographs of the past certainly aid this process, triggering and stimulating feelings, fantasies and memories.

As we shall subsequently see, photographs can serve to help us learn to manage our load through facing the internalised 'monsters' of the past. The therapeutic process aims to free the patient from some of the bonds of the past – but obviously the pain will not be forgotten. Past images, irrevocably frozen into memories and often confirmed and clarified by the photograph, cannot be eradicated or erased. They will live on in the mind forever.

However, therapy enables such traumas, once they are made conscious, to be worked through, so that the patient can carry the burdens of the past more easily. Such burdens then become lightened and cease to interfere with everyday living.

The importance of the patient–therapist relationship

The patient will be able to expose the innermost self only in a safe, trusting and secure atmosphere. Thus it is necessary to emphasise the importance of the relationship between therapist and patient. The therapist needs to 'be with' the patient in every sense, accepting, warm and non-judgemental.

If the therapist is able to be empathic and understanding, to establish rapport and a secure therapeutic alliance, the patient will learn – in time

– to trust the therapist with intimate and private feelings in an atmosphere of safety and confidentiality.

The patient will be encouraged to free associate, to share thoughts and feelings in an open and uninhibited manner, without fear of interruption or judgement. Then, the patient's own, inner material will emerge; personal symbols and images will surface, ready to be explored and understood in therapy.

Photographs very much aid the establishment of this relationship; as they are shared, the beginning of a dialogue is encouraged, one that emerges from a seeing into a patient's world as well as a hearing of their story. They can be used to promote a real therapeutic conversation, helping to forge a bond between the therapist and patient.

The search for meaning

The subsequent quest for insight and understanding is of central importance to the therapeutic process, for, whilst the firm foundation of trust and empathy is a crucial prerequisite for therapy, this alone is not ultimately enough to facilitate real change. What must ensue is a search for meaning. Some kind of sense must be made of the host of cryptic messages that we receive from the patient, fitting them into some sort of cohesive whole.

So we ask: what lies beneath and beyond the presenting problems, the symbols, metaphors, symptoms, feelings and behaviour? Can we discover in them patterns, common threads that will help us make sense of the myriad of enigmatic images and signals from the unconscious? The search for meaning involves an understanding that all these signs are not random, indiscriminate products of chance, but indicators of deeper, intensely meaningful life-themes, with significance in the past and the present. We search for some order and coherence out of the seemingly disparate parts, whilst still, of course, maintaining a tolerance of the paradoxes within that order.

Photographs offer an extra dimension in the search for meaning – we are able not only to listen for meanings behind our patients' words – we can look for them in their photographs. The verbal communications are complemented by the visual ones. Lost, long-forgotten meanings, shrouded in fear and resistance, can emerge through the study of our personal pictures.

Working through

Photographs may also assist the process of working through. This is another essential element in therapy and involves continual reconstruction of past events and repeated confrontation of old blocked feelings and attitudes in order to gain new insight into the self. Working through helps to strengthen understanding by re-viewing the same issues again and again. Yet, each time there may be some small difference to be perceived in the patient's response; perhaps some new snippet will emerge, to cast a new light on old themes, or maybe a slight shift in attitude will occur, barely discernible, yet significant in the scheme of things.

As part of this process, photographs are often brought back repeatedly, with the same ones re-explored time after time, in the hope of gaining a different view, a greater degree of self-knowledge. Patients may feel that they are continually going over the same ground, getting nowhere, yet each time they face resistances and blocked areas, they are attempting to move nearer to awareness and clarification.

For many of us, in our everyday lives, photographs, especially old ones, are perused again and again in a similar fashion, almost as if they provide us with a way to work through our feelings and confusions about ourselves and our relationships. Perhaps this is also an attempt, unconsciously, to review how one's attitudes to the photograph have changed, and to use the photograph as a measure of change inside the self.

The therapist's role

Let us now consider the role of the therapist in terms of the therapeutic use of photographs. In relation to this, questions emerge: what is the therapist's function in helping the patient to look at photographs? How is this done? In what ways can she enable an exploration that will increase the understanding of what lies beyond the two-dimensional images?

No 'right' way

In addressing these questions, it is necessary to begin by emphasising that there is no right way to interpret a photograph. There is only the individual patient's way. Interpreting someone else's photograph is like trying to explain another person's dream – it is solely the associations of the dreamer that are relevant. The patient alone knows what the picture means internally and what it holds in terms of personal memories and associations. The therapist therefore assists patients in their photographic exploration in a way that does not involve an imposition of her own views; she helps them to explore photographs through her attitude of encouragement, her facilitative skills and her interest, whilst all the time following the patient's lead.

An insistence by the therapist that she knows the 'right' meaning of a photograph would be a denial of the uniqueness of the patient's feelings and experiences. It would also replicate the kind of defeating pedagogical approach from which many people have suffered in childhood, the primary (though perhaps unconscious) aim of which has seemed to be to convince children that they cannot know their own mind and that they are therefore in need of the advice of someone 'wiser' than they.

Being with . . . sometimes silently

In order to remain facilitative and open and to avoid such attitudes, the therapist need only be sure that she has an understanding of the power of the photograph to keep meanings secret, an ability to enable their discovery by the patient and an astute awareness of unconscious processes. From the start, she also needs to be quietly aware of her own counter-transference reactions.

Counter-transference refers to the feelings and reactions of the therapist in response to the patient and, frequently, to the photographs. These images may trigger strong responses in the therapist that are a reaction to their power in the patient's life. It is very important that the therapist takes note of the impact of the patient and the photographs on her – such feelings are positively useful to the therapist in gaining a real understanding of the patient's world by actually feeling into it herself through her counter-transference responses. (However, the photographs may also trigger some feelings in the therapist that are her own, personal ones, and reactivate memories that are about past issues in the therapist's life. Then it is important that the therapist is able to differentiate between herself and the patient – in Chapter 8 this issue will be more fully explored.)

Initially, as we have seen, it is important that the therapist has the ability to 'be with' the patient, free from pressure to do or achieve, whilst the pictures are perused. The therapist needs to avoid disturbing her patient with her own thoughts and ideas.

Wordsworth potently expresses the necessity to resist the temptation to over-analyse, or to make clever interpretations which can spoil special moments:

> Our meddling intellect
> Misshapes the beautious forms of things –
> We murder to dissect.
>
> Enough of science and art;
> Close up these barren leaves;
> Come forth, and bring with you a heart
> That watches and receives.
>   (Wordsworth, 'The Tables Turned')

It is through such 'watching and receiving' that the therapist stays with the process, using her intuition to sense the patient's needs. There may be many times when the patient can only be in silence with the photographs. Many people find verbal expression difficult; they may be choked with emotion, too stunned or traumatised to utter a word, or very afraid of what they might hear from the depths of their own being. Some feelings, thoughts and memories may seem too terrible to be spoken.

Yet there is simultaneously a need to reach beyond the paralysing fear; a wish for contact and communication. The photograph can offer an experience of being seen in a relatively safe way, of being heard and not heard, in that it speaks visually for the patient.

Just as people have a right not to share photographs, so they have the right to be silent; the value of such a wordless experience can be enormous. There is still a silent communication, and a safety that is created through the use of a photograph that provides containment and a preparation for words. It is sometimes also easier to recall incidents in visual terms than verbally, for words may be too disturbing.

Elizabeth had found that her words often produced negative or dismissive responses in others, and she felt isolated and unheard. She had, some years ago, been very overweight, but was now slim. However, she was beset by old fears and negative feelings about herself and her body. She felt that only a photograph would be able to convey her massive size. Eventually she did pluck up courage to bring one to the session spontaneously – and the fact that she was able to do so had positive implications about the therapeutic relationship. It meant that Elizabeth had *shown* me a part of herself, and her past, about which she felt ashamed and secretive – for her it was important that this part of her could be acceptable.

In time she managed to bring in more pictures of her former self into therapy, and those soundless images told of the acute pain and embarrassment she had experienced as a hugely overweight teenager.

There were many times when we sat in silence for a whole session, sometimes with her collection of photographs upon her lap. She would stare mutely, solemnly, into the silent, unseeing images that were so painful to her. Occasionally, she would look up at me, her deep, meaningful gaze speaking of measureless pain; but there were no words. It was not difficult to understand the message in her eyes. She needed both the space to contemplate the photographs and the experience of being with them – and me – in quiet reflection. During subsequent, more verbal, sessions, Elizabeth told me that, after the silent times, she felt some relief: 'Most people have not been able to hear my words when I speak. You showed me that you are prepared to hear not just my words, but also my silence. That was very important to me.' This kind of silence felt productive and healing; the therapist needs to be aware, however, that sometimes silence can be frightening and she may need to help the patient through it.

A unique kind of language is discovered when the photograph is shared in therapy. There is a kind of visual conversation; a communication through looking that needs no words.

Two people contemplate photographs in silence: much is communicated;

sitting quietly together, engrossed in the looking, they are mutely acknow-ledging feelings of mutuality and respect. The silent conversation speaks volumes about the value of being with, being there, as a solid, reliable presence for another human being.

Whilst some patients may want to express their feelings in another medium such as painting, others may be too afraid, depressed or restrained to risk this activity. Creativity can in itself be a stressful experience, and the ready-made photograph provides a short-cut when image-making seems too difficult. The sharing of photographs in this instance offers a gentle encouragement to verbal expression, a relatively unthreatening way to help someone to connect with and express feelings. Sometimes, how-ever, these can only be communicated non-verbally.

A criticism that is on occasions levelled at psychoanalysis has been that it is primarily most appropriate to those who can verbalise and conceptualise in a lucid and clear way. Perhaps the introduction of the use of photo-graphs in therapy may mean that it becomes a little more available to those who are not easily able to articulate, or indeed be physically creative.

Not knowing

In therapy, as patients grapple with their memories, it is important that the therapist is able to wait, without needing to know: 'The experienced therapist . . . has to make an effort to preserve an adequate state of not knowing if he is to remain open to fresh understanding' (Casement 1985: 4).

This state of 'not knowing' is a crucial one in relation to the use of photographs in therapy. The therapist's attitude of quiet acceptance, her unspoken assertion that everything the patient brings is meaningful, will communicate a faith in the process of looking at photographs that will contain the patient's doubts and fears. The message thus given is one of belief in patients' autonomy and a conviction that it is they who know what their photographs are about, not the therapist. In being free from pressure to achieve or to be result-oriented, the therapist provides a strong presence for her patients, encouraging them to stay with the experience of not-knowing, perhaps in the silence of contemplation.

Sensitive interventions

In time, when the patient is ready for words, the therapist must facilitate a real looking at the photographs by means of sensitive interventions. She needs to consider carefully the kinds of statements and questions to make, so that these may pinpoint the areas that are likely to produce insight. Working gently and with understanding, the therapist will avoid over-exposing the patient to the possibly unsettling images. She will need to ask the questions that may facilitate a real looking into the photographs, remembering that 'a wise man's question contains half the answer' (Ibn Gabirol from Rosten 1977: 483).

We can interpret this statement, in terms of the photograph, as meaning that, whilst the therapist does not actually know the answer for the patient, her experience of working with photographs will be a guide towards the areas that will lead to the most enlightenment. She will be looking for process within the patient's photographs, recurring, repeated patterns that may indicate aspects of personal behaviour and relationships. As will be further explained in Chapter 5, one photograph may not on its own be relied upon to indicate a habitual pattern. It may have captured only a quirky expression or position, which may not be characteristic or usual.

However, if the patient has a series of pictures, all depicting similar repeated patterns, then these are more likely to be indicative of something significant. Illustrations of how photographs can be used to highlight and trace such patterns will be given in Chapters 5 and 6. Detailed attention will be given there to the importance of positioning in a family or group picture, and what this may be indicating at an unconscious level.

With practice, the therapist will develop an ability to identify these significant themes and elements in her patients' photographs that will help them towards insight. Looking at photographs in a therapeutic way certainly becomes easier with experience. The increased confidence and creativity that such experience brings, will inevitably generate innovative and special ways of photographic looking for therapist and patient.

The therapist will then feel secure enough to make hypothetical sugges-tions, based on how she perceives the pictures, whilst at all times checking these out with the patient, and never imposing her own perceptions and views. The patient may confirm or deny the therapist's perceptions – either response will help the therapist's understanding of her patient and aid in the joint process of discovery.

Facilitating play

It has been interesting to observe how photographs help to lessen people's self-consciousness. In a trusting atmosphere, they will inevitably reach a stage of reduced inhibition. Within the safe constancy of the therapeutic relationship, they can be encouraged to feel free enough to 'play'. This involves therapist and patient joining together to use images and words, symbols and metaphors from the patient's inner world in an imaginative way. The therapist needs to demonstrate how to play with these images, both verbal and visual.

Many people cannot feel relaxed enough to play with images and fantasies. Often, as children, they have not been permitted to ponder and dream, to 'stand and stare'. They may therefore have drifted into anxious escapism, rather than experiencing the letting go of tension that is a prelude to playful creativity. Perhaps they have been given too many regulations and their own play has been curbed by adult intervention.

Playing in therapy will aim to help counteract these restrictive influences, enabling the growth of spontaneity. Such play can effectively be centred around photographs, with the therapist learning the patient's special 'language', the personal images that are most symbolic and meaningful. These become a sort of shared secret. This increases rapport, for the therapist has been permitted to enter the patient's private world and to gain an understanding of personal symbols.

Thus as patient and therapist interact, they create their own rules of play. In addition, the photograph gives them a unique opportunity: they can play with time. There is a playful suspension of disbelief as a picture-show of the past is recreated in the present.

The photograph can also be used to stimulate fantasies – perhaps the patient can be asked to imagine it coming to life.

What would the feelings be if this were to happen? How would the people in the picture act, what would they be thinking, feeling or even saying? How do their imagined words reflect the patient's inner scripts, those messages from the past that play and replay deep inside us? Perhaps patients could project themselves physically into the photograph, imagining where they would be if they were actually in the picture, and how they would feel, in there.

Being aware of timing

Within the sessions, the importance of timing can not be overestimated; it links with waiting, in that a patient will be able to explore photographs therapeutically only when the time is right. As will be seen in the next chapter, any pushing from the therapist towards the premature exploration of photographs will be counter-productive. It is important to have trust in the wisdom of the patient's unconscious; it has a protective function, knowing its own solutions and revealing them only at its own pace.

An example of this may be seen in the case of Michael, who had come into marital therapy some time after his wife had begun. At the beginning, he had been very afraid to remember or explore any of his childhood experiences. He had said, 'Can't we do this therapy without looking at my childhood?' This was, in effect, a strong 'Keep Out!' warning. As trust increased, he became less and less resistant, safely looking on and pensively absorbing his wife's impressions – photographic and verbal – of her own childhood.

After some weeks, feeling less threatened and certainly more relaxed, Michael said that he was finding therapy enlightening and that looking at the relationship had almost become secondary to personal discovery. He began to link some of the lonely feelings he had in the present to his past, but had some difficulty in remembering anything other than an image of himself as king of the castle in his family, in a kind of exalted, yet isolated position.

He was now clearly communicating that he was ready to explore the past, just as he had made a definite initial statement to the contrary. Unconsciously he knew the time was right, and I wanted to respect this. He subsequently produced more striking verbal images of his past, and my suggestion to bring photographs enabled him to produce a plethora of meaningful visual ones.

Being aware of space

Photographs in therapy also act as a bridge, a link between two separate people and their worlds. They connect them, span the space between, a space that can be full of creative possibilities. The therapist needs to manage this space with sensitivity, and to understand that it represents symbolic issues in the relationship. She must ensure that she is psychologically close enough to empathise and respond, but sufficiently distant to maintain a detached and objective view, in order to help the patient to gain a new perspective on old images.

The issue of physical space is also relevant to the therapeutic use of photographs. One cannot share these images without physical proximity; there is an inevitable drawing near. Often, the album is opened or photographs are displayed in a giving way, with the intention of sharing visual intimacies with the therapist. The atmosphere becomes less formal and more trusting; there is a moving together emotionally as well as physically. Whilst therapeutic boundaries are maintained, the space between the patient and therapist will adapt to and absorb the movement and fluctuations within the therapeutic relationship.

The bringing of photographs to therapy

Frequently, photographs may be brought into therapy spontaneously during the initial stage of therapy. Sometimes, they are produced by the patient at a later stage.

They assist the therapist in her learning about the patient, and the family history. Photographs will help the patient to assemble a kind of chronological life-history book, thus enabling both self and therapist to gain a fuller life-picture, past and present.

We have seen how Elizabeth, the patient mentioned above, produced the photograph of her former overweight self of her own accord; people sometimes do bring photographs in this spontaneous way, or allude to them freely without any prompting from the therapist. During the process of therapy, as memories slowly return and old scenarios are re-lived, certain photographs are often intuitively recalled. Like the spontaneous bringing to therapy of dreams, photographic memories will often grow out of the process naturally.

Sometimes long-forgotten images suddenly materialise in the patient's consciousness. The fact that certain photographs should enter the mind at such times is hardly surprising; we have seen in previous chapters how photographs play such an important role in the course of our lives in terms of documentation and memory-preservers.

It is usually during childhood reminiscences that photographs are remembered. They are then often described in detail, and their description can provoke considerable emotion. John, who had been physically and emotionally abused as a child, was trying to convey the sense of deprivation with which he grew up. Almost involuntarily, a childhood photographic image of himself floated into his mind. He saw the child he had been – eczematic, puny, afraid. Visualising the photograph, he described the child as having 'no body.' This image was vividly recreated internally and he wept as he saw it.

There was a prolonged silence as he grappled inside with the disturbing picture. We waited. It was important to empathise with his pain, and, when he was ready, to help him search for the meaning within his statement, and beyond the remembered image. We 'played' with the words 'no body' and discovered that they could be heard in three ways, all of them relevant and pertinent to his feelings at the time: he was painfully thin, there was nobody there to help him, and he felt like a 'nobody'. This image produced many more painful memories, and helped John to get in touch with his past suffering – and to begin to convey this.

Motivations

Patients bring photographs to therapy, both literally and symbolically, for many reasons; it is very important that the therapist looks at the bringing of the photographs in the context of the whole of the therapy, and at what this may be indicating about the patient.

There may be a positive need to strengthen memories, get in touch with feelings, recreate the past, expand consciousness of self and other. There may be a wish to at last hear – and see – the child who still exists within them, perhaps ignored and unheard until now. Often, needy children are labelled as attention-seeking, rather than attention-needing. The photograph offers another opportunity to face the child within, and give that child a voice.

However, a photograph may also be produced in order to avoid difficult feelings – as a kind of diversion or defence. There may be an unconscious resistance to facing hidden, conflict-laden aspects of the self. Whilst it is these very conflicts which have brought people into therapy, paradoxically, the fear of confronting them may produce resistance to their therapeutic exploration. Then the photograph may be used to present an image of self or other to the therapist that is narrow and one-sided, reflecting the internal splits in the patient. The picture can maintain and perpetuate these splits by fixing them into an image that represents an almost absurd simplification of reality.

Initially, the therapist will accept the partial image as reflective of the patient's fear and resistance; it will serve as a way into subsequently understanding the whole picture. With further encouragement and empathy, the patient may be enabled to complete the incomplete images, present a more whole picture to the therapist. This may be done verbally, as therapy progresses, with the patient perhaps bringing additional photographs to add to the partial images at first selected.

The freezing of the image can also sometimes arrest the process of recollection, stunting and retarding memory. It is important not to become attached to one particular photograph in a way that hinders a wider view. This further highlights the paradoxes inherent in the therapeutic use of photographs – they can present us with past realities or make us blind to them.

The therapist needs to be aware of the possible motivations for the showing and bringing of photographs, especially if the material is produced in some way to manoeuvre or control the therapist, or to avoid or distract from difficult material.

In this context, and by way of example, Winnicott, in his paper on 'The Manic Defence' discusses the bringing of photographs into therapy by his patient, Mathilda, aged 39.

> The patient now produced what is called a Polyfoto of herself. Her mother wanted a photo of her and she had felt that if 48 small photos were taken (as by this method), one or two might be found to be good. Also this method corresponds to a hope of putting together the bits of breast, of the parents, of oneself. I was asked to choose which I like best, and also to look over all the 48. She intended to give me one. The idea was that I was to do something *outside the analysis*, and when, instead of falling into the trap (a few days before she had given me warning of such traps), I started analysing the situation, she felt hopeless, she said she would not give the photo to anyone, and that she would commit suicide. We had had a good deal on the subject of looking as giving life, and I was to be seduced into a denial of her deadness by looking and seeing.
>
> (Winnicott 1958: 142)

Winnicott further comments that the patient '*felt it more real for me to see her photo* (a 48th of her) than for me to see her herself' (Winnicott 1958: 142).

After this incident, Mathilda begins to get in touch with the pain in her lonely inner world, to face the loneliness of being herself, rather than to avoid it. Winnicott adds: 'I have quoted Mathilda chiefly to illustrate the feeling of unreality that accompanies the denial of inner reality in manic defence. The Polyfoto incident was an invitation to me to get caught up in her manic defence instead of understanding her deadness, non-existence, lack of feeling real' (Winnicott 1958: 143).

As with any powerful therapeutic tool, there is potential for photographs to be used as avoidance or perhaps to manipulate the therapist. This need not be regarded as negative or destructive, for it will provide fertile material for exploration. The bringing may represent attempts to please, divert or distract the therapist; all these actions are in themselves communications and need to be considered as part of the patient's whole story. The therapist needs to be aware of their meaning in the full context of the therapy, and of the patient's life, past and present. Part of the therapist's task, therefore, when photographs are brought or mentioned, is to have a scrupulous understanding of the multiplicity of motivations and feelings that spur the patient on to bring photographs into therapy, and to be able to use this understanding effectively for the patient through sensitive interpretation.

When can the therapist introduce the subject of photographs?

When there are spontaneous allusions to photographs, or when they are actually brought into therapy, there is communicated a natural wish and, generally speaking, an ability, to use them in some way as part of the therapeutic process. In the absence of any mention by the patient about photographs, there may be times when the therapist feels that it might be appropriate to introduce the subject herself.

Therapists will, as they become more adept at using photographs and in the natural course of the work, devise specific ways of asking for photographs that reflect their personal style and also the needs of the individual patient. There will inevitably be differences in approach; it is most desirable that therapists discover the ways of working with photographs that suits them.

Some therapists introduce and use photo-therapy from the beginning of the work with the patient. Akeret (1973) asks his patients during the initial consultation if they have photographs with them – if they do, he asks them to take them out and look at what makes them particularly important. This seems a most valuable way of working, because it immediately selects out and identifies the significant photographs – and through these is most likely to highlight the personal themes that may be most significant to the patient. Having explored these, he later asks specifically for photos to be brought.

My personal preference in terms of suggesting work with photographs is to wait and be fairly selective about the patients to whom I put forward the notion of photographs in therapy. The medium does not suit everyone – nor, indeed, does it suit every therapist. With our knowledge of the immense power of the photograph to confront and sometimes distress, it is crucial that we assess the patient's suitability for such an approach.

Assessment for photo-therapy

Most of the accepted criteria for assessment for psychotherapy will apply to assessment for photo-therapy. The therapist will, for example, want to see that the patient has an ability to express thoughts and feelings, and a wish and motivation for insight and change from within. There will be some potential to think in a psychological way, to understand that past experience influences present feelings and behaviour, to make some sort of relationship with the therapist, to respond to interpretation. She will note whether the patient has enough ego strength and ability to cope with the stress of the therapy experience, and does not have defences that are too brittle, nor acts out inner pain in an overt way.

However, if the patient is to work with photographs, there will need to be, in addition, an ability to use visual symbol and metaphor creatively. Most people have some aptitude for this; photographs especially, have a quality of universality and familiarity which increases the appeal of photo-therapy and provides a safe container for creativity.

Whilst the majority of those assessed as suitable for psychotherapy can benefit from the therapeutic use of photographs, they obviously vary in terms of the depth to which they can relate to visual imagery. A few people do not find it possible at all to use visual symbol and metaphor imaginatively and creatively; they cannot trust themselves or others sufficiently do so (Plaut 1966).

In addition, it must be emphasised that photo-therapy is not a suitable medium for those with rigid defence systems; often the power of the vividly disturbing images can increase resistance. One needs to feel as sure as possible that the patient can tolerate the frequently graphic reflections and unsettling implications that result from photographic exploration. Photographs can precipitate and trigger depression, which may be a very necessary part of the process for a patient who is ready and able to face such inner pain, but too overwhelming for one who is not.

The therapist uses her sensitivity and experience, both generally and specifically with each patient, to decide whether the patient could cope with, and benefit from, the use of photographs. This assessment for photo-therapy may not necessarily occur at the beginning – it may emerge, reflectively, later in the therapeutic process, growing out of it, as it were. The patient may not be ready to look at photographs at the outset of therapy, or be sufficiently trusting of the therapeutic relationship at this point. Perhaps there is not yet enough courage or ego-strength to face personal photographs and all they have to reveal. Timing, as will be seen in the clinical example in the following chapter, is of crucial importance.

Is the patient ready?

My current practice is to let the subject of photographs emerge, as far as possible, out of the patient's own material in therapy, as it did in the aforementioned case of Elizabeth. If it does not, one can wait until there is some indication of the patient's readiness to respond to some mention of them. It seems to me vital that any such suggestion by the therapist should take the form of a considered response, one that is rational and measured, based on a synthesis of thought and intuition. It must be attuned to the patient's personal themes – both on a symbolic and a literal level – and should never be an impulsive reaction that merely represents the therapist's own interests, theories or needs.

Photographs are a useful adjunct to whatever process patients have initiated for themselves, after they have begun to overcome initial resistances. They will serve to enlarge and enhance the flow of therapy, to illustrate and magnify memories and impressions, and to stimulate further material. They are not a way of prodding the unwilling or resistant patient to remember, feel or imagine and must not merely be introduced as an active response to, or avoidance of, difficulty.

If the patient is experiencing stuck or lost feelings, there may be a need to stay with these and with the pain, so that their meaning can be explored and understood. This exploration will take place within the context of present and past experience. A 'flight into photographs' by the therapist may be a part of her counter-transference response, reflecting the patient's internalised pressure; the real impetus for further exploration always needs to come from the patient, with help and support from the therapist, who follows the patient's lead.

Patient-leads

What, then, are the patient-leads, the cues to listen for, that would induce the therapist to suggest the bringing of photographs? How can the therapist gauge whether the patient is ready? It is important to notice when the patient naturally uses visual imagery in the material brought or, alternatively to observe the response to the therapist's encouragement to visualise.

The patient may make spontaneous comments like: 'I am picturing myself as a child, standing alone in the middle of our big garden,' or: 'Let me give you a picture of my father/husband – I want you to get an impression of his size . . .'

The therapist needs to keep a sensitive ear out for such clues. Sensing the appropriate moment, she might venture to respond: 'Maybe you have a photograph from that time . . .', and then, if the patient does have, she can help with an exploration of the photograph in the patient's mind.

If the remembered photograph is, for example, of the patient as a child, the therapist can stimulate the patient's visual imagination, inspiring 'play' with the fantasied image, to explore it in 'full colour'. Encouraging a patient in this way will help stretch and develop the creative imagination; an ability to respond to this kind of visualisation is a good indicator for further work with photographs. It is quite possible to utilise such a remembered photograph in therapy without the picture ever being produced; indeed, it may be that the photograph is never brought into therapy in any other way.

At times, however, such discussion, perhaps over several sessions, may be a prelude to the actual bringing in of a difficult photograph. Some encouragement from the therapist, at the appropriate moment, may mean that the patient is enabled to bring in the photograph that is most troubling. The therapist only suggests the bringing – and must leave it to her patients ultimately to decide if they want to follow the suggestion through.

Tim, in therapy for about six months, had great difficulty getting in touch with any of the feelings he had had as child. Sensing his readiness, I wondered if he could picture the child in his mind. He looked at me with some puzzlement at first, and then, wordlessly, his gaze diverted away from me and upwards to the sky through the window, as if looking into a place – and time – far away. Slowly, a dim picture emerged within him, which he was able to describe, haltingly, for our exploration.

After a while, I asked him if he had any photographs of himself as a child. He said immediately that he had just one, a professionally taken picture that he liked very much. We focused on the remembered photograph for a while, and then I ventured to suggest that he might want to bring it. He seemed uncertain, excited by the prospect, yet afraid of the exposure. He reflected at that point that he could never have contemplated telling me before about this photograph, and certainly could not have considered bringing it. That would have been too intimate, he said, and before then, he had not felt able to let me in.

Today, it felt as if he was beginning to bring his inner child to me in therapy. He was then able, for the first time, to describe to me this 'perfectly composed' child, who never made a mess – that would not have been tolerated. He saw that this reflected his difficulty in bringing messy emotional material to therapy, for fear that I would not be able to tolerate it. Really it was he who could not cope with that idea.

In the following session, he 'forgot' to bring the photograph, but he had had a dream about photographs. He dreamed that he had found several bright, colour photographs of himself and his siblings, and they gave him startling new insights; subsequently, however, on waking, he could not remember what those insights were. He felt that the dream and the forgetting expressed his ambivalent feelings about therapy; it also high-lighted his mixed feelings in relation to facing his photographs and the emotions connected with the images they portrayed. The session was spent exploring his dream – and this ambivalence – and making links between past and present feelings in relation to revealing himself to others.

The next week, he was able to bring the picture into therapy, and it formed the basis of further work on himself. There was thus a kind of preparation, a softening of the anticipated impact of the photographic image and its painful associations through the groundwork of the previous sessions.

Having identified one important photograph, patients may feel inspired to think of other photographs that are interesting and may spontaneously bring many more pictures to therapy. If they do so, it is very important that the therapist allows them to make free choices about the kinds of photographs they will bring.

Once the photographs have been brought after a period of preparatory discussion, it may be also relevant for the therapist to note just how much they coincide with the pictures that the patient had described. How far do the selected photographs correspond to the patient's narrative? How much do they fit the therapist's imagined picture, in reponse to the patient's descriptions? Is the therapist surprised at the photographs, or are they the way she imagined them to be?

This kind of enquiry may reveal the extent to which the patient is ascribing feelings or characteristics to the person in the picture, which in fact belong to him or herself; this is the unconscious psychological mechanism known as projection, a way of disowning uncomfortable feelings by attributing them to others.

When the photographs are eventually brought to the therapist, they may also provide her with an indicator about the assumptions which she may have made about her patients, their families, their backgrounds. Does the experience of actually seeing the photographs reveal that she was forming faulty opinions based upon her own fixed ideas?

Selection of photographs by patients

Considerable attention needs to be given to the way in which patients select the photographs to bring into therapy. Whether patients have brought photographs from the family album, or have taken them them-selves, whether they bring them of their own accord or are following a suggestion from the therapist, their choices must be seen as an important focus for discussion and exploration.

Selecting people 'out'

These choices may have been made in a deliberate way, or unconsciously. What has made the patient decide to bring those particular pictures, and maybe even more importantly, what photographs have been omitted? There is a paradoxical significance in the photographs that the patient does *not* select to bring to therapy – these indicate more than meets the eye and such omissions should be noted and actively brought to consciousness in the course of therapy.

Depending on individual patterns of facing or avoiding problems, the patient will choose to bring – or to leave at home – the pictures that best reflect principal internal themes. Even when the patient has not actually created the photographs, the choices made will, unconsciously or consciously, serve as symbols of what is significant, representing internal aspects within the patient's hidden world. It is therefore most important that the therapist is aware of the unconscious motivation behind the patient's selection process.

Alan chose to bring a number of photographs into therapy – mostly of himself at various stages in his life. He mentioned casually that he had 'literally hundreds of photos' at home. In response to this throwaway remark, I asked him if he could think about the selection he had made, and especially about the photographs he had not brought. Alan pondered for a while, and then was himself surprised to discover that, when choosing the photographs to bring the previous evening, he had deliberately not brought any pictures of his father, without fully realising why. Then he reflected: 'He's always intruded, I want to keep him out of here, I want to be in the limelight, be the king. He always overwhelmed me, related to my friends and pushed me out; I'm pushing him out now.'

Alan was simultaneously telling me something about the past, the present, and the here-and-now of the therapy situation. He did not want to have his father intrude between *us*, even in a photograph, so powerful was the parental image. He was actively taking control in keeping him out and was also avoiding facing the internalised image of his father, represented by the external photographic image of him. His anger towards his father, previously completely repressed, began to surface as he examined his own motivations in selecting him out.

At that point, however, he began to look more closely at his photographs and he did find that he had, in fact, brought just one photograph that showed his father – but very much in the background, and hardly discernible. In this picture (Photograph 7), Alan was posing proudly with his brother in the foreground, and behind, one can just perceive father's head, through the back window of a car, straining to see what is going on. It was as if, unconsciously, Alan had brought the picture of his father that most safely contained and controlled him, for he looked quite squashed and restricted, securely framed within the small back window.

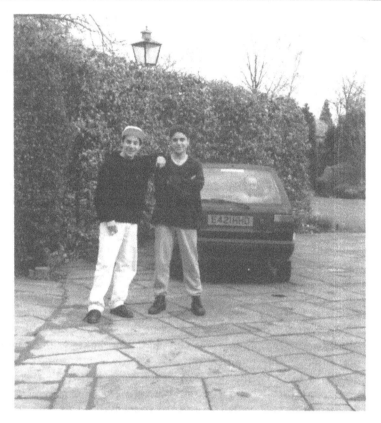

Photograph 7
Posed by models

Subsequently, Alan did manage to bring more prominent images of his father, and to get in touch with powerful feelings of envy, rage and pain in relation to him. He was also able to understand how his father's extravert qualities, as embodied in these pictures, represented denied and repressed aspects of himself that were, in fact, replayed in his own marriage.

When the therapist is asking about selection, she needs to maintain a respectful attitude to the photographs the patient does present and, where appropriate, to ask gently about those that have not been brought and perhaps look at why they are being avoided. She can then explore the basis on which censoring has been done or selection made. Additional focus may be given to the reasons for liking or disliking certain photographs, and why some pictures are especially significant.

The process of selection in itself can reveal considerable valuable information: did it pose a struggle, a dilemma, and if so, why? If the patient has been selective, what sort of information would the other photographs have yielded, and how would the present therapy session be different if those had been brought? Sometimes the patient conveniently 'forgets' to bring the photographs, or loses them. In such instances, it is important to see the forgetting and the losing as material for therapy, and to explore them and make connections in the context of the patient's whole story, past and present. Perhaps they are indications of a fear of finding the photographs in the fullest sense of the word.

Manner and order of presentation

The therapist can also take note of how the photographs are stored and presented. Are they gathered into untidy bundles, a little torn or crumpled, in no particular order? Alternatively, are they neatly, or obsessively, arranged in albums, complete with explanatory labels and captions? Whilst one must resist over-interpretation of such issues, they may possibly be indicators of aspects of the patient's inner psychic organisation.

Once in the room with the therapist, the selection process continues: the patient then chooses the order in which the photographs are to be presented and looked at. There will also be significance in terms of the degree of attention given to particular photographs: some are perused in depth, whilst others are lightly skipped over. When photographs are quickly set aside, it may sometimes be appropriate to point this out to the patient, for it may indicate a resistance to staying with a particularly difficult or disturbing image.

The process of showing

At times, the patient may appear embarrassed when first showing personal photographs; after all, this is likely to be a new experience, and there will be feelings of uncertainty about its outcome, or how the therapist may respond. It is common for the patient to feel at first that the photographs are inconsequential, that they hold no meaning, are unimportant or trivial – both to self and the therapist. This may also be a defence against discovering the truth in the opposite – that the photographs are, after all, a treasure-house of meaning.

Some people need to share their photographs immediately; others may be more tentative, wanting to peruse the pictures alone, with the therapist present, but not directly sharing the experience of looking. I have known people who stare fixedly for long periods at a picture, holding it tightly to their chest in furtive perusal, perhaps in silence, or interacting verbally with me. There needs to be no pressure from the therapist to share photographs visually – the fact that they have been brought does not mean that photographs *have* to be shown.

People have a right to keep some photographs to themselves, unexplored. It seems important not to turn even the page of an album without permission – after all, its owner may only want to share specific pages. If there has been an opening of an album, this must be seen as a symbolic opening up of the self, and there must be sensitivity to this fact. Some photographs may feel too private to be shown, now or ever, or the therapist's physical approach may be threatening and be experienced as an intrusion.

It is vital to remember to let the patient reveal the chosen pictures in his/ her own time and space. Only when – and if – there is some indication of readiness, will the therapist lean forward to see, as the photograph is offered for shared exploration.

The symbolic journey of therapy is one of discovering an inner self, traversing from the known into the realms of the unconscious. There may be the prospect of a rough crossing, and so it is crucially important that the therapist is aware of the significant risk involved in the bringing and sharing of pictures and is sensitive about attitudes towards personal space and boundaries.

Uncertain and apprehensive at the outset, it may be that the patient will start to select the more superficial photographs as a way of 'testing the water'. The therapist needs to empathise with this, valuing each picture for itself, and to wait until the patient feels confident enough to examine the more difficult ones.

Transference issues

There may be, on the other hand, an attempt by the patient to hand over all the photographs to the therapist with an unspoken message of 'Well, I've brought them – and I've seen them all before – now you interpret them.' It is important that the therapist does not collude with this request for instruction and that she gently encourages the patient to begin to look in his or her own way.

People often want to be told what to do in their wish to find an all-coping parent. Most often, they will repeat childhood relationship patterns in their reactions to the therapist, re-experiencing with her many of the feelings, attitudes and behaviours that originated in responses to important people from their past.

The therapist's aim is to help patients face the disappointment and grief involved in the realisation that there are no parents and that real solutions lie within the self. This is disappointing because many have longed for salvation from an all-knowing figure who will make everything right for them. It will not be possible to let go of this fantasy until patients become a little stronger and more sure of their personal power, through experiencing a new, enabling and encouraging relationship in therapy.

In her firm yet gentle refusal to act as if she were a parent, or to take sole responsibility for photographic interpretation, in her giving back to patients their responsibilty for themselves, the therapist begins to demonstrate that they are no longer powerless children, but adults who are respected for their autonomy and individual views.

This act of handing back responsibility shows that the therapist neither intends to deny her patients' rights to self-determination, nor to collude with fears that they cannot help themselves. The hope is that people will develop, through the relationship with the therapist, faith in themselves, new and strong internal relationships that are nurturing and self-supportive.

The therapist begins to facilitate therapeutic looking . . .

If the patient feels overwhelmed or inhibited by the number of different photographs, it may be necessary for the therapist to be initially facilitative by indicating the kind of photographs that might be most therapeutic. So the therapist might say: 'I am wondering which of your photographs might be particularly meaningful for you, perhaps in terms of some of the issues we have been exploring up to now. . . .'

Larry, in his thirties, responded to this with particular immediacy; having looked at his photographs rather blankly at first, he now was able to select instantly a photograph of himself at 5 years old, on holiday with his father, framed by the majestic portals of an old Italian hotel. What was most noticeable about this picture was the austerity of the atmosphere, which reflected the relationship, and also the distance between the two. Although they were holding hands, their arms were almost outstretched, so that the picture seemed full of space, lacking intimacy.

The photograph immediately identified an ongoing problem for Larry. It highlighted the ambivalent feelings he had towards father, resulting in a difficulty in relating to men and an intense feeling of inadequacy compared with others. My intervention had given him a necessary signpost and helped him quite quickly to make an introductory, and most meaningful, selection.

It has been interesting to note that such a comment frequently produces an instantaneous and definite response in patients, as if, consciously or unconsciously, they have come to the session with the most relevant photographs already selected. Patients simply need the right trigger from the therapist to enable this to surface, so that these photographs can be produced for initial exploration. They soon learn how to choose from amongst the photographs those that are pivotal to an understanding of self and significant others. Gradually, the original awkwardness in talking about the pictures, frequently expressed in comments of not knowing where to start, gives way to a process of free and personal selection.

Because the therapist does not start the selection process, but encourages

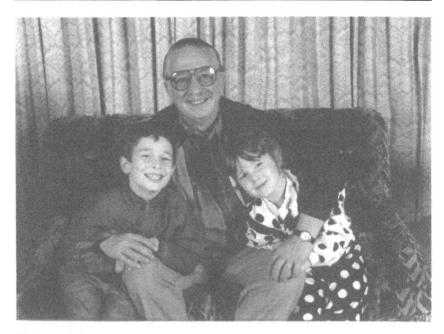

Photograph 8
Posed by models

the patient to do so, she is following the patient's agenda, not her own. She may very well have experienced at the beginning of the session a feeling that nothing very much was going to emerge. There may have been a temptation to collude with the patient's assertion that the photographs are not going to be useful, and to set them aside. At the beginning of every session and beyond, the tolerance of the doubt and even scepticism that the patient feels is most important if the atmosphere is to be set for a therapeutic experience.

Some initial considerations

Once patients have selected their photographs, the therapist's interest will focus initially on scanning them for important details. It is relevant to ask who has taken the picture, however, because this may very much influence the attitudes of the subjects.

To illustrate this point, take a look at Photographs 8 and 9. Photograph 8 shows a man with his two grandchildren upon his knee. They all look happy; the children's mother is the photographer and they smile at her cheerily. Now take a second look. Can you spot anything else in this picture to comment on or detect any deeper issues? On closer exploration, you may notice the way in which the man is holding the children, how his

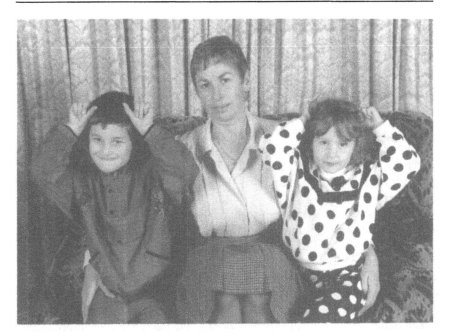

Photograph 9
Posed by models

hands are grasping theirs in such a way that they cannot move them – he is controlling the children, making them pose for the camera.

Now let us see what is happening in Photograph 9. Here are the same children again, this time on their mother's knee, and the picture is being taken by the woman's father. Spot the differences. . . . Can you guess their feelings about him? Observe the children's gestures and expressions, the fixed, angry look in the woman's eyes, the angry, ambivalent, mere trace of a smile in contrast to her father's broad beam.

As the woman perused the picture, she felt herself becoming irate and upset at the memories it provoked. Her verbal account confirmed that whole family was very antagonistic to the photographer; her mixed feelings about having her father take her photograph are written all over her face. The father was experienced as strict and aggressive, and his daughter felt anger and hate towards him for his childhood treatment of her. Notice also in this second picture, the increased freedom the children have with their mother. Encircled by her protective, yet totally unrestrictive arms, they obviously feel safe enough to act out their (and her) feelings towards grandfather.

When such photographs are brought to therapy, the patient can be asked for thoughts and feelings about the photographer's motivations in taking the photograph, and the therapist can help the patient to explore fantasies about the possible attitudes to different photographers. If the patient had taken the photograph, and thus had had the power and the control, how would the picture have been different?

Subtle photographic messages

The therapist will, at this stage, be looking out for oblique and intricate messages in the photographs, subtle elements that may reflect whole areas of meaning and interaction, perhaps hitherto unnoticed. There will be a search for contradictions, incongruities, symbolic and metaphorical content; her keen eye will be caught by the details that are different, arresting and unexpected.

As therapist and patient pause and linger over each individual print, there will be discoveries that cannot be made at first sight. The photograph is closely perused with a sense of heightened awareness, enabling a detailed examination of every part of it. It will be scanned to perceive the smallest nuances, gestures and expressions, the most subtle minutiae of human behaviour that can prove to be so symbolic and yet may have escaped initial cursory glances.

The patient will be encouraged to identify the people in the pictures, and to reclaim memories about them, exploring the feelings and thoughts associated with everyone in the photograph, noticing their postures, body language and expressions, their relationships to each other and to the self. The picture will be thoroughly scanned for 'giveaway' clues that may betray hidden feelings and thus facilitate greater knowledge and insight.

It may be that one particular photograph is found that symbolically encapsulates a family problem. Such a picture will be seen in Chapter 5, (Photograph 13), and may be compared to a hologram, which is a photograph whose fragments reflect the whole picture. In Photograph 13, parts of the picture express something of the wider history and interaction of the family.

Finding holograms, patterns and reflections

We may also find holograms within therapy. It is interesting to consider that, within every individual session, there are many symbolic holograms. Aspects in each session will mirror the wider story, just as the fragments of a hologram reflect its whole. Thus core themes in a patient's life will be reflected in the many small ways of relating to the therapist, in body-language, facial expressions and gestures. The medley of symbols and images within photographs will also explain and highlight broader issues if the therapist is able to be sensitive to their presence.

Thus, when the patient is looking at photographs in therapy, the therapist does not focus exclusively on them. In order to see a fuller picture, her awareness stretches beyond their boundary, extending to all that occurs within the therapy room. She will also watch out for the photographs that produce the most intense feelings and memories in the patient, either positive or negative.

Perhaps each whole therapy session, too, can be seen in terms of the hologram. As the session continues, I have often noticed that there emerges a structure, an overall form, a natural pattern that may be more apparent at some times than others.

After the initial waiting, as meanings surface and become explicit, there is a kind of climax to the session that involves some insight and perhaps new understanding. As the process of looking at photographs develops, there is always a sense of growing excitement with the emergence of new insights. Towards the close of the session, this understanding continues to be processed and integrated, in a reflective and thoughtful way. The session now has a kind of pattern of its own, a structure, which gives it shape, a beginning, middle and end. It can be seen to reflect the whole structure of the therapy over weeks, months and years.

In the following chapter, it will be shown how several of Jane's photographs vividly expressed and reflected larger life-themes. We shall also see how Jane used her photographs in therapy, struggling with the painful images they portrayed, eventually to attain enlightenment.

Chapter 4

A clinical example
Jane

. . . part of the built-in interest of photographs, and a major source of
their aesthetic value, is precisely the transformations that time works
upon them, the way they escape the intentions of their makers.

(Sontag 1987: 140)

Within the following pages, I describe in detail one person's experience of
using photographs in therapy. Throughout the weeks, months and years
of Jane's therapy, the presence of photographs added a most important
third dimension to a painful, yet ultimately fulfilling, personal journey.

The case of Jane will serve to illustrate many of the theoretical issues
described in the Chapter 3, and to introduce yet more. In its initial stages,
this material also illustrates the usefulness of photographs in helping to
define and isolate important themes and issues beneath a presenting
problem.

THE THERAPY

Jane, an attractive, slim woman of 47, described herself wistfully as 'just
a housewife'. She had been married since she was 19, and had two grown-
up children: Michael, aged 20, who lived at home, and Joanne, 23, who
was married with a young son. Jane felt very protective towards her
children, and was especially worried that Michael might inherit her
problems. She saw her marital relationship as – 'generally good – I trust
and love Peter dearly, but I am mostly a "yes-person" to him, especially
when he loses his temper'.

Jane had been taking Valium for over twenty years and had been
referred by her psychiatrist, in an attempt to help her off the medication.
She was very anxious and felt upset that she was to be encouraged to stop
the Valium. Her self-esteem was low and her fear of making mistakes
meant that she never took any risks; life felt hollow and meaningless.

Jane was tormented by memories of having been let down by a
constantly depressed father (now dead), who took to his bed for days on

end, and a mother who did not have time for her. Only her older sister, Marilyn, in spite of her own childhood illnesses, had been able to offer Jane a degree of emotional support. As an adult, Marilyn suffered from a severe depressive illness, which disturbed Jane greatly; it meant that Jane also felt debilitated when her sister was ill. Anything potentially enjoyable, like family parties or holidays, was spoilt for Jane in her present life by her anxiety and fear.

Feeling that she was inferior and uneducated in comparison with others, she was especially troubled by the notion that she hardly read a novel, lacking concentration, whereas *everyone* else read 'several books a month'. Jane was highly conscious of her appearance, and always made sure that she was dressed immaculately. Her ability to choose beautifully stylish clothes for herself was the only area in which she felt confident. She never confronted anyone, for fear of making them ill, and tried to please everybody, turning the angry energy upon herself.

Jane was quite resistant in therapy at the start, having a very harsh superego, which made her extremely self-blaming. She was taking responsibility for everyone, and at the same time very strongly pressurising me to take responsibility for her, desperately wanting instructions as to what to do to remedy the situation. Jane seemed to have only a little insight into what all this had been about for her in her past, and a dreadful fear of looking at any of her own inner destructive impulses.

After the first few sessions of therapy, she began to relax a little, and to make one or two links between her past life and her present feelings and behaviour. As she returned weekly to therapy, however, she became more anxious to find a solution from me, and to be given guarantees that the therapy would 'work'. It felt as though a kind of pressure were building up inside her.

In session ten, she talked of envious childhood feelings towards her sister, who had a new dress for a wedding, whilst Jane did not. It was at this point that I asked if there were any photographs of the wedding; she said there were and yes, she would bring them. Jane duly brought a pile of photographs to the next session, which she had secretly taken from her mother's house. She had been surprised to find that there were more of her father than she had thought, and that she was with him in some of the pictures.

She was able to do a little work with the photographs, selecting one that showed her when on holiday with her family – she was arm in arm with her father, and he looked very depressed and sad (Photograph 10). Looking at the picture, the memory of how holidays were inevitably spoilt by father's illnesses was awakened. As a result, she was then able to make an important link for herself – she saw in the picture the source of her inability to enjoy holidays in her present life – she realised why she spoils them for herself now. The vital black and white evidence of the photograph

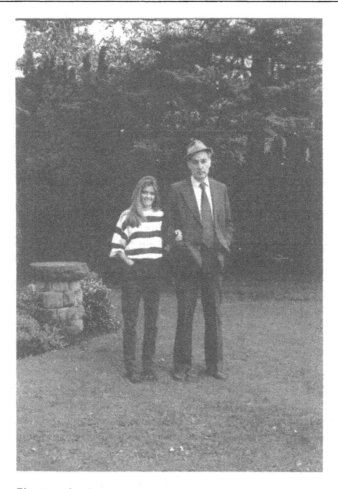

Photograph 10
Posed by models

helped her to make the clear connection between past and present that was crucial to her subsequent understanding of her adult dilemmas.

However, it then all became too much for her. She grew highly resistant, asking impatiently 'What am I supposed to feel? . . . Why do I have to do this to get better?'

As she said these words, she took out a picture of her father in morning suit (Photograph 11). He was going to someone else's wedding.[1] It was a source of massive distress for Jane that he had subsequently been unable to attend her own; looking at the photograph created considerable disturbance. Deeper exploration of her anger and sadness in connection to this picture of her father was too overwhelming. Her feelings began to

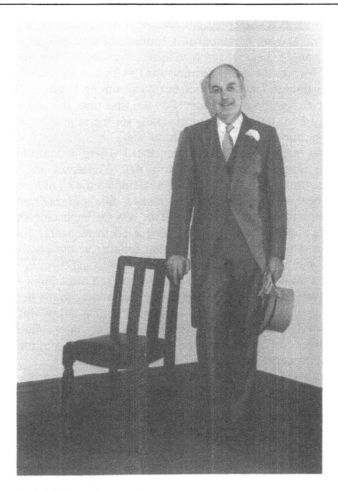

Photograph 11
Posed by a model

surface in an agonising way; father was re-experienced, the emotions recalled. It was almost as if one could feel his presence in the room and all that it symbolised for Jane. Quickly he was put away amongst the other snapshots, securely 'lost' in a disordered heap of pictures, piled in safe disarray.

At the next session, photographs in hand, she was very low. She felt that everything was going wrong and she could not see how photographs – or therapy – could possibly help. She was obviously angry with me. She said that she was only coming to therapy because others said that she should and had felt very down after last week.

I wondered whether my suggestion about bringing photographs had felt like a request that she could not refuse. It had always been difficult for her to risk another's disapproval, either through pleasing herself or expressing anger. Jane reflected on this. After some silence, she then said, quite firmly, that she really did not want to look at the photographs, but wished to discuss feelings about her forthcoming holiday. This was an important change point for Jane. For the first time she was saying what *she* wanted from therapy, without waiting for me to give her some advice or solution. She was showing me some anger.

Jane had really grasped the notion that she was in control of her own destiny in terms of therapy and this was a different and therapeutic experience for her, for she had never contemplated such autonomy before.

In the next session, she appeared clearer. She told me, quite firmly: 'I don't want to look at photos yet.' This was an important and symbolic statement, and the beginning of a long road to recovery. Subsequently, she explored many of the feelings that looking at the photographs had triggered, but without them in front of her. Keeping them in view during this period would have been too confronting, too threatening. It was as if she had glimpsed the worst of what she had to face, found herself unable to do so, put it away, and then started again at a less difficult point. Unconsciously, she had known she was not ready to encounter the most painful issues 'yet'. She spent the next few sessions exploring some very important concerns that emerged spontaneously for her.

Then, at session twenty, she showed a readiness and a need, albeit rather contrived and controlled, to 'face things'. She continued:

> I did not know you then, when I first looked at the photos. I do now. I want to face my wedding album and look at the feelings, and cry and then put it away. . . . I'll be honest with you, if I had the pills, I'd take them, to hide the pain, but I haven't, so I'll do it this way.

Jane had learned that she could have some control in the session, and that she could risk trusting her own feelings and thoughts, without disapproval – or contradictory advice – from me. She began to take responsibility for her own process in therapy; previously she had so much wanted me to give assurances and point the way.

The photographs that Jane had selected initially – showing father on holiday and in morning dress, helped to pinpoint two specific and symbolic issues: her feelings that good things would be spoilt, especially happy family occasions, and her anger and pain at not having people there for her when she was in need of care and comfort. These two pictures represented general childhood feelings of loss and emotional deprivation, of not being seen, heard or given enough parental attention.

Subsequently, Jane was able to select more photographs that symbolised and identified past problems with which she was still struggling.

As Jane determined to face her pain through the pictures, she chose one

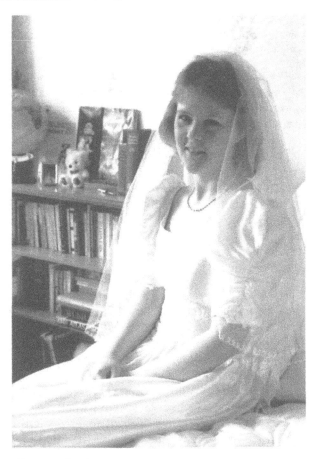

Photograph 12
Posed by a model

particularly distressing photograph from her wedding album (Photograph 12). It showed her in the bedroom she shared with her sister, just before she had left for the ceremony. She was sitting on the bed, in her wedding dress, smiling. In the background I had already mentally noted some important symbols: rows of books, arranged on shelves.

Jane gazed at the picture, and spoke with sadness in her voice: 'Look, in the background are my sister's belongings.'

I waited. She did not comment on the books. I ventured: 'I can see that there are books, behind, on the shelves. . . . I know they've been a difficult issue for you. . . .'

Her expression darkened. She spoke quietly, not without bitterness: 'Yes . . . I suppose they sum up all my feelings of inadequacy, compared with her, my sister. I always felt a lack of equality with her. I was inferior to my sister where education and reading were concerned. Those books were all hers, I had none.'

This tendency to measure herself against others seemed to have its origin located right there in the picture; the photograph graphically signified the source of the troubling present-day problem. It is thus most important to look at a picture not only in terms of the subjects in its foreground, but also to explore the background closely. Similarly, objects and settings, as well as people, may yield a wealth of information and serve as a basis for understanding.

Jane's graphically symbolic book image, frozen within the past, was revivified and subsequently enlarged into a new understanding in the present. It expanded into an awareness of the link between her past and present feelings of not being as good as other people, and it gave her an insight into the roots of her problems in the area of reading, which had long troubled her greatly.

'I suppose that's why I have difficulty reading today, and why I feel inadequate when I see others reading books', she said, 'It probably started with my feelings about my sister.'

That felt like a big realisation. I said: 'It sounds like you are seeing the connections between your feelings today and those of your childhood though the photograph, sort of making links . . .'.

She looked at me, relieved. A little braver now, she risked sharing some difficult feelings: 'You know, I can also feel envy when I see those books. . . . I can still feel it, now. Marilyn seemed to get everything, all the attention, all the fuss from my parents, because she was so often ill, and she was the cleverer one.'

The pictures then helped her to reach some previously forgotten memories: 'Those books weren't all – she seemed to have all the new stuff – clothes as well, whilst I got her cast-offs. I just think that my parents didn't see me, or my needs. In their eyes, I was OK, the "happy" one. . . .'

Jane was subsequently able to recognise the guilt she was carrying for the envy she felt towards her sister; this had, in fact, made her over-solicitous of her sister's welfare in her present relationship with her. She saw how she had taken on the role of protector in a family that could not cope and she repressed all the anger over this, turning it upon herself.

As Jane became more aware of the wider setting in the picture, painful memories were stirred up. Haltingly, she described how she could hear the awful groans of her father in bed in the next room. She began to recall feelings towards people who were not actually in the photograph, but elsewhere in the house at the time. The photograph enabled a recall outside its own parameters, triggering fuller memories than it was able in itself to visually record. The picture stimulated Jane to auditory memories as well, so that she could hear the sounds in the house at the moment the photograph was taken, over twenty years earlier.

Spontaneously, Jane proceeded to put the photograph into its time context, by describing what had happened immediately before and after the picture had been taken. This is a vivid way to recollect whole memories from a snapped moment. Jane had become deeply engrossed in the photograph, so that the surrounding time was involuntarily recalled, permitting a strong recreation of the original experience. What began to emerge from the captured time-fragment in the picture, was a full extract, a complete scenario from this continous, painful life-story.

Just before this photograph was taken, Jane had gone into her father's room, in her wedding dress, and asked him to go to her wedding. But he was too ill. Jane saw herself, minutes later, smiling, in the picture, blocking out feelings and the sounds, determined not to let all that spoil her day. But now, as she looked back, she felt all the pain that she could not let herself feel at the time. She remembered that, after the picture was taken, she had left for the church. Now, turning the page of the album, she found a picture of herself there.

At this point, she began to cry freely, profusely, because her father was not in that photograph. She wept for herself as she had been, longing for father to be at her wedding. The photograph, as well as presenting her with reflections of her wedding, also emphasised the incompleteness of the experience for Jane. Paradoxically, it faced her with an image it did not portray – that of her absent father.

At the end of this particularly emotional session, Jane asked to leave the album with me; this testified to the power of photographs and the need to have me literally and symbolically hold all the pain, which may have felt unmanageable alone.

As Jane explored her photographs weekly in therapy, she gradually began to get more in touch with the child she had been. She now felt a great need to cry for that child, who had put on a brave face throughout her life and had held back feelings. It was still difficult to release tears, especially when there was another person present. However, she found she was able to cry and release sad feelings when she looked at the photographs.

As Jane slowly grew in confidence and strength, she began to use her photographs in a more actively experimental way. Between the sessions, in her home, with the family photographs in full view, she started to write letters to her parents, not to be posted, but for her own inner work on connecting with the powerful parental images internalised since childhood. From time to time, she stopped her writing to focus on the visual images; much repressed anger surfaced, as she addressed the people in her photographs and a deep bitterness emerged that surprised her. Exploring these letters in therapy, and looking at how let down she had felt by her parents, she began to realise that her own expectations of perfection – for herself and in relationships – were unreal. This lowering of expectations was one of the main areas of learning for Jane and a main theme in this case. She saw the huge burden of responsibility she had tried to carry as a child, and how she continued to do so in her present life. She now recognised the impossibility of that role, past and present. As she freed herself from these internal bonds, she was able to be stronger in her external, real relationships with her family and friends. She now had less need of her medication to suppress the feelings, and this was reduced at her next visit to the psychiatrist.

The strength that Jane gained through confronting her family in therapy through the medium of their images in the photographs, became generalised to the outside world, so that she felt more easily able to manage the relationships in reality. She began to be able to risk showing her needs to her family, and to stop allowing herself to be emotionally walked over. She had also made a spontaneous shift from a more passive looking at her pictures into a phase of active work that perhaps indicated her readiness to move towards termination – symbolising her move out of the therapy situation into the 'real' world.

She continued of her own accord to bring in large numbers of old family photographs, now addressing herself principally to her mother. She repeated to her: 'There were two of us!' Beginning to connect freely for herself past and present experience, she instructed me to take out the photographs for her at the beginning of each therapy session. She began to face and work through feelings of hate and rivalry towards her sister and also to realise that her expectations that therapy would totally cure her were unreal, that the scars were there for good because she could see them in the photographs, and that therapy was not about eradicating them, but about helping her to live with them. The photographs provided powerful visual evidence, confirming a painful past.

That summer, Jane was able to have a good holiday for the first time, without sabotaging it for herself with negative thoughts. She was starting to shed some of the feelings of responsibility for others, especially her sister. For when her sister had been ill, she had felt that her life was ruined, and she, too, became ill. At this point, she began to use the photographs to grieve over the sister she once had, and needed so much. She also expressed anger through the photographs about her sister's illness, wishing that her sister would just die.

After discharging some powerful rage, she was able to be firmer with her family, and some anger was expressed outside the therapy in response to requests to take on responsibility she did not want. She was beginning to stand up for herself. She decided to finish therapy in six months time, when the birth of her second grandchild was imminent, feeling that that was symbolic, of new life, for her, too.

Soon after this, Jane took out again the photograph of her father in morning dress, the picture that had been so disturbing for her at first. This time she looked at it in a different way; therapy had enabled her to reconstruct and reframe this picture. She now said that it would have been better if father had been able to rage, especially at her mother, who always put him down. She was able to see that, like herself, father was angry inside, becoming ill with all the emotional repression. Jane had used the photographs in therapy to recognise family patterns. That was the first time she had ever looked at his illness – and perhaps her own – in any other way than organically. With encouragement from me, she was able to let herself talk to him directly in the picture about this.

The photograph permitted a talking on two levels: Jane was speaking to the image of her father, and also addressing a part of her self, for they had both shared the same problems. The image represented both a past external reality and an aspect of Jane's present internal conflict. The dead father no longer existed in reality; but he was very alive inside the self. She was talking to him and to herself, but only the inner 'father' heard. In revisiting an old conflict through this photograph, Jane learned to reframe it within the context of her new understanding about herself and her inherited patterns. She was now more able to see her symptoms in a symbolic way and to link them to her past and present emotional states. Perhaps, her husband, too, in his frequent bouts of anger, had been expressing unconsciously aspects of Jane's repressed rage, on her behalf. Jane began to be able to stand up for herself more in her marriage, and to feel less dominated.

Subsequently, in the ensuing sessions, Jane was able to continue her more active work with photographs, releasing much anger and tension through such activity, and reaching a cathartic peak of emotion. She used the pictures in a more tactile way; her handling of them grew more confident and she began to manipulate and use them to suit her needs. She selected two photographs of a family get-together, when she was about 13. Both photographs showed Jane with her parents and sister. She hesitated before speaking. 'I feel mixed up – angry towards my sister, yet I do not want to hurt her. But I also do.'

I knew that the photograph, a rich medium for working through such paradoxical feelings, might be useful here. I risked: 'I wonder if you can have both those, using the photograph – hurting and not hurting. . . .'

She looked puzzled. My comment had been ambiguous, perhaps confusing. Then, suddenly, she made her own sense of it. There was an excited gleam in her eye. 'You mean I could rip the photos?'

I had not specifically suggested that, nor had I actually thought of it. But she had quickly picked up and elaborated on my statement in a way that suited her. She stared at one of the photographs a while longer, then started to look more angry than I had ever seen her. I felt a mounting tension in the room, a kind of slow crescendo.

'We always had to share everything. Even that dress I'm wearing, that was my sister's.'

Decisively, she ripped off the dress, and the bottom part of her sister's body, leaving her head. 'Now maybe you can see why I'm so fanatical about nice clothes.' She had made this link for herself here, wih no prompting from me.

'I was always expected to share everything with Marilyn.'

'And perhaps now you are sharing her illness?'

'Yes – I hadn't thought of that, but it's true, isn't it. . . . But then I always did share her illnesses, as a child. . . . My Mother always expected me to share everything with her and now I can't live my own life and get away from her illness. I wish I could tell her how bad I feel about all this.'

'She is there, Jane, in the picture. . . .'

She paused, looked a little frightened and began to cry. Gaining courage, she addressed herself loudly to her mother in the photograph: 'Let me go! I do not want to share her illness!'

She repeated this several times, with much passion. Then, through tears, she looked up at me, and explained: 'I was never there for them, they only saw Marilyn.'

'And you have felt some envy and some anger about all that . . .'

'Yes, I am angry . . . and with Marilyn. . . .' She faltered then, changed direction, appearing to feel guilty, responsible again: 'Well . . . if only she'd get better, I do want her to get better, you know, and to have everything nice. . . .' She grew silent, eyes lowered. Moments of flatness descended upon us. The crescendo was lost.

'Those are real, strong feelings and sentiments that you've expressed here a lot', I said. 'There have also been other feelings, that come alongside them, perhaps less reasonable, less rational, that you felt when Marilyn got all the attention. . . .'

She did not respond to this with words, but it seemed to free something, for without more ado, she ripped off her sister's head in both the photographs, and then her body, adding with some glee: 'I like destroying things.'

Then she looked again at the pictures. She saw that on them both she was left standing next to her parents. She put aside one of the photographs, leaving her parents together in that one. She picked up the other, and tore her parents apart from each other, saying 'These two should never have got married.'

She looked again at the other snapshot. She saw herself, standing next to her parents, just the three of them. Her sister lay ripped up, on the floor, at her feet. We looked at what was left. I reflected: 'That looks different now, you on your own with your parents, without your sister there.'

She looked up at me, angrily dissatisfied with my comment. 'But, can't you see, they still wouldn't see me! They'd be so busy mourning the loss of Marilyn that they still wouldn't see me!'

I hoped then to encourage her to take the power over the internalised parental figures: 'It seems really difficult to get yourself seen or noticed in that family, even now, when you are in control.'

She then ripped off the figure of herself on the picture where she had left her parents together. It was almost as if her unconscious mind had planned to leave them together in this picture so that she could use it later. Having torn herself off, she firmly and deliberately positioned the part that showed herself as a child directly in the line of her parents' gaze. She addressed herself to them, loudly: 'See me! . . . I'm here! . . . (Pause . . .).'

She straightened herself in her chair, staring into her parents' eyes. Then she smiled, and glanced at me. 'It looks like you have been seen. . . .', I said.

She replied, triumphantly, 'YES!'

This was a powerful and emotional session for Jane, one that brought to the surface many deep and repressed feelings about her family relationships. As she ripped the photographs, she dropped all the torn off fragments round her feet; at the end she gathered them up and threw them in the wastepaper bin. It felt as she if she were throwing away old patterns, chiefly involving the need to share others' pain in a self-sacrificial way.

Symbolically, she has thrown off the internal pressures represented by the images of her sister and she had for the first time 'made' her parents see her. She said afterwards: 'I have difficulty destroying things'; it will be noted that she said the opposite during the session, appearing to very much enjoy the destruction. In a later session she revealed that she had been told as a child, she thought by mother, never to tear up photographs, because it was thought to bring bad luck. Then she added: 'But I want to – I like it!' It felt as though there were some freedom in doing the tearing, from parental messages and ties, as well as ambivalence about her own destructive impulses.

In the following sessions, over the remaining months of therapy, Jane continued to confront the power of her sister's illness, which of course echoed that of her father and reflected aspects of herself. She looked at more photographs of herself and her sister together. Tearing off the images of her sister, she said: 'I don't want her to die, but I do especially want to get away from her interminable illness. I want to separate us a little.' This statement did not only refer to the external separation of the two sisters, but chiefly to the internal separation, the internally binding sister from whom she was struggling to separate.

Whilst she kept the parts of the photographs that depicted herself, she told me that she was throwing away the damaged pictures and fragments, saying that doing so made her feel better. Many of these were of her (internalised) sister, and the discarding of the heavily symbolic images was accompanied by talk of separation and refusing to take on responsibility for others any more. The external, physical treatment of the photographs potently symbolised aspects of Jane's internal processes, for she was now demonstrating a readiness to lessen her rigid hold on the inner damage.

Gradually, as therapy neared its end, she began spontaneously to take the photographs back home, leaving only a few with me. Those remaining were of herself as a child, mostly with father, a few with mother. Perhaps she was giving the child that she had been a chance to be alone with her parents. As the quantity of pictures in my care became smaller, it was as if their lessening numbers represented her decreasing need for transitional links with me. These photographic points of contact were slowly becoming less functional and necessary.

Jane had asked for a phased termination; in view of her difficulty in separating, it felt important to manage our ending with sensitivity and care, without it feeling as if we were abruptly cutting off from each other. Thus, we arranged to meet for a follow-up session in two months' time, so that Jane could move gently out of the therapy relationship, testing the water, returning to share with me how she was getting on. This follow-up would allow Jane also to look back and review her therapy, having had some space. I wondered privately how she would manage the leaving, given that one of the main themes of her therapy had been around separation.

During the first follow-up session she did not look at the photographs, but she still wanted to keep them with me. She was not quite ready to have them back; the reprocessing of them before the final handover was not quite completed. We arranged another follow-up, some three months later. It was during that session that she said that she really did not want to be back and did not really feel the need to come. Things were very much the same in her family, but she definitely seemed to have a different attitude. Her sister had become ill on Jane's return from her last holiday – and Jane had realised that, unconsciously, her sister had wanted to spoil her holidays, out of envy. She had worked that out for herself. Jane also seemed more accepting of mother's attitude to her, and was no longer trying to change her, nor expecting approval or recognition. She seemed to be living with her difficulties and focusing on the changes in her life that were making it much more bearable, not on the problems that remained.

She suggested in a sort of resigned way that we should make another follow-up appointment. I had noted that she had not wanted to come today, and wondered whether she felt she 'ought' to return. This comment seemed to bring her considerable relief – in that I did not expect her to come again – she had needed to feel encouragement and acceptance to leave, without guilt or recrimination.

She said she would take back the remaining photographs. I retrieved them from the drawer; holding them on her lap for a few moments, Jane began to look through them. I wondered what she intended to do with them. She said that she had thought about throwing them away, but then had dismissed that idea. She had decided to take them home, but not to dispose of them.

'Maybe one day, I'll creep into my mother's house and quietly put them back where they belong. They are hers, not mine. All the photographs I have at my home were taken after my marriage – and they signify happier times. Perhaps now I want to leave the unhappy memories with my mother. They belong to her, not me.'

As the session drew to a close, Jane got up to go, saying 'Thanks . . . I'm not very good at goodbyes.' She tucked all the photographs back in their envelope and put them in her bag. We said a simple goodbye, and she left, for the last time.

EXAMINING THE PROCESS OF JANE'S THERAPY

Beneath Jane's low self-image and fear of displeasing others was a store of repressed anger that had originated in childhood. Through the therapeutic relationship, the lack of judgement and atmosphere of acceptance, she was able to risk showing feelings that had hitherto been repressed and stifled. This gave her a new and different experience. As an adjunct to the therapy, the photographs helped Jane to confront her past, regain some memories and to allow hitherto unconscious material to come to the surface of her awareness.

Within the safety of therapy, she risked expressing feelings, giving voice to her own views and wishes, letting her true self emerge. The paralysing fear of her destructive impulses lessened because she was able to risk acknowledging them and, through her photographs, to express them safely.

The therapeutic boundaries of time and place, together with the reassuring containment of the photographs, provided Jane with the safety to push beyond the limits of usual acceptable behaviour. She was able to risk breaking the habitual social conventions that had previously kept her fettered and to experiment with new, more open, ways of being.

Through the insights that followed this cathartic self-expression, Jane was able to reduce her need to placate and please people constantly, for she saw how she had taken on responsibility and guilt for the pain of others, denying her own needs. She began to gain a sense of her individuality, an awareness of her separateness, initially from me as a person in therapy, and then from the world.

Jane also lowered her expectations of her self and others, largely because she gained a more realistic awareness of the limitations of therapy, which could not make everything perfect for her.

Through examining in more detail aspects of the process of Jane's therapy, which lasted for sixty-two sessions, it is possible to see exactly how useful the photographs were in helping her to identify and subsequently emerge from her emotional problems.

The transference and counter-transference

From the beginning, in the transference, I was to Jane the all-knowing mother for whom she longed; I had the key to the relief of her distress. I was also the withholding mother who would not give her that key. She wanted to turn me into an active problem-solver who would put it all right for her.

My suggestion that she bring photographs was perhaps a mistakenly active response to this transference. I acted out my counter-transference, instead of letting this tell me more about how Jane had felt in her past; for Jane had spent her childhood feeling responsible for finding impossible solutions to the interminable problems that surrounded her.

I was mirroring something about Jane and the messages she was giving me, and perhaps also showing something of my own pathology here – a rather omnipotent wish to 'get it right'. (Here is a similarity between therapist and photographer: both can simultaneously reflect in their mistakes aspects of themselves and their subject/patient, and these mistakes can make a strong statement about the relationship between the two people.)

However, through this experience of acting out my counter-transference, I was able to understand and feel the real pressure within Jane's inner world. With a clearer view, I was able to be a strong presence for her, responding but not reacting to the frustration that she felt at not being directed. This helped Jane eventually to begin to take responsibility for herself, to realise that I was not going to solve things for her, so that she could discover the potential within herself.

Earlier in the therapy, Jane also experienced me in the transference as the mother who expected her to be strong and not to cry; for a long time she found it hard to look at me and show emotions in the room. Yet we have seen that she was able to cry when she looked at the photographs. This illustrated the fact that they must have made a considerable difference in terms of the relationship in therapy, enabling her to feel freer to express difficult feelings. The album served as a 'kind of shock absorber' (Searles 1960: 79), a containing object onto which she could focus her pain and tears. It also functioned as an intermediary between herself and me, whom she experienced in the transference as mother intolerant of her tears.

As she reproached the figures in the photographs, she was also making a communication to me, through the images. Jane's difficulty in crying in front of me was reflected in, confirmed and explained by her parallel reaction to the images in her photographs. There she faced a family whom she experienced as unable to cope with her vulnerability. Her attitude to the pictures reflected the transference to me as someone who could not abide her tears. Gradually, as she became more integrated, she began to risk more direct expression of her feelings to me and to move from fantasy into reality.

As we have also seen in the chapter about paradox, photographs can offer the chance to work on both a reality and fantasy level, to integrate inner and outer. By crying into her album, risking tears in the room and occasionally sneaking a look at me, she began to discover that she would not be stopped or discounted in her sadness or her anger. There began some resolution of the transference. Through the safe medium of the photographs, Jane was somewhat freed from the fear and guilt that would have been involved in confronting me directly, or in addressing the real people represented by the photographs. Whilst she was able to do both these eventually, the photographs, used within the therapy relationship, initially provided the kind of 'nursery' conditions that were necessary to nurture and protect the fragile, growing inner child.

Resistance

We have seen how, having taken an initial look at her photographs, Jane grew resistant to further exploration, having glimpsed the extent of her pain. The barriers had begun to be eroded in therapy and, as a natural part of the process, resistance set in. Whilst Jane consciously wanted to get better, there were also fears and doubts about coping with change and recovery. So, in therapy, there is often resistance to insight, as the patient is threatened by the prospect of new and painful awareness and learning. The very paths to enlightenment are unconsciously blocked.

In stark monochrome or flagrant colour, photographs confront us with realities we may not wish to observe. They face us directly with past trauma and with troubling issues in the present, helping us to recognise the areas that we wish to avoid.

Only after the trust and the therapeutic alliance had been built up in the therapy was Jane able to make the choice to confront her photographs again. Up to then, it obviously had not felt safe enough to do so. She needed to find the courage really to confront the painful images. When she did risk this again, she began by approaching her photographs in a rather organised and planned way, but this soon grew into a more spontaneous kind of looking and feeling.

Once she really faced her photographs, they did help Jane's resistances to be decreased, providing a way into her unconscious pain, stirring memory and feeling. They served as reminders, and ways of correcting assumptions, so that initially she was surprised to see so many pictures of her father and of her childhood self by his side. Photographs such as this can remind us of a forgotten reality, and present us with surprises about our own lives.

Leaving photographs with the therapist

Whilst Jane was working with her pictures, her request to leave them with me between sessions was most significant. It reflected both the power of the photographs, and also her trust in me as therapist to contain the difficulties symbolised within them, and to hold onto these whilst she was working through them.

If the therapist can demonstrate an ability to manage such issues for the patient, then she will help the patient to feel secure enough to continue the struggle. Perhaps there will then be some resolution of the difficult issues, within the supportive atmosphere of the therapy. Eventually, the photographs can be returned into the patient's possession, once this process has taken place, and when the disturbing images have been managed, defused and thus made safe.

Whilst we have seen that photographs are potent symbols, what is done with them is also symbolic, and great attention must be paid to how they are handled by patient and therapist. One patient said, on giving me his photographs until the next session: 'I'm leaving part of myself with you.' The photographs were mostly of himself as a child, a child whom he found it difficult to nurture or connect with, and whom he experienced as 'troublesome'. This was the part of himself he left with me. The therapist needs to take any photographs that are entrusted to her firmly and with care, showing the patient where they will be kept, perhaps emphasising that she has a drawer or cupboard for photographs, and that they will continue to be safely stored there.

When the patient returns to the next session, however, it is important that the therapist has not taken the photographs out, prepared for the patient. This would take away the patient's freedom to begin the session spontaneously and would represent an imposition of the therapist's expectations. The patient may not choose to look at the photographs that day; perhaps they will remain safely untouched in the therapist's room for many months.

The search for meaning and insight

Through personal pictures, patients are helped to get in touch with and clarify the real issues behind their symptoms and presenting problems, and to learn more about the roots of their present-day dilemmas. It will be observed that, almost from the start, Jane's photographs served to distinguish and identify problem areas.

At the outset, Jane had no conscious idea of where her problems lay, but was plagued by an intense anxiety, haunted by faceless ghosts that would not let her rest. Through the medium of the photographs, she was more quickly able to identify the core troubling issues in her inner world, so that they could be named and recognised as the real source of her problems. In this way, photographs can also aid the therapist in assessment and diagnosis.

Jane's photographs also helped her towards a more interactional view, rather than remaining isolated and inward-looking, trapped within a vicious circle of self-blame and deprecation. As therapy progressed, she began to see the family context in which her problems had arisen; her photographs offered her images of the 'other', stimulating thoughts and feelings about relationships, widening understanding and insight.

The fact that photographs permit a view of the past in the present allowed Jane to link childhood experience and present feelings and behaviour in a way that produced insight and some resolution of painful, stuck feelings. In linking past to present through the images and recognising repetitive family patterns, Jane was also able to perceive implications for the future. She saw that her sister was handing on some destructive family patterns to her children, like the repetitive spoiling of family holidays and the perennial fear of them going wrong. Jane was proud that, through her own awareness, her children were free of such fear, and she felt sad that her sister's seemed to have become caught up in it.

In addition, photographs enabled a differentiation for Jane between the then and the now, a realisation that, whilst some situations and attitudes around her may have remained the same, *she* had changed, she was not the small helpless child trapped in a sick family. The photographs also helped in the bringing of old rules and patterns to consciousness, so that these could be assessed within the context of her present life.

Generalising from the experience: the power of the image

It was evident that Jane was able to confront images of her family through the photographs in a way that was ultimately releasing. This prompts the question: how does working with an image of a person in therapy help or affect the relationship with that real person or situation?

It may appear to some people that this use of the photograph is unreal, and nothing like confronting the true-life person. Yet such is the power of the photograph to recreate and symbolise the inner or outer difficulty that the patient most often finds that troubling issues have genuinely been faced.

There *can* be a generalising from the experience with the photograph; real inner change, rippling through the patient's psyche, produces further transformation in many areas of life. Action will naturally follow a genuine change, one that is truly based on a synthesis of new experience and fresh insight. It does not have to be prescribed or planned. This emphasises the strength of the psychoanalytic approach: change is facilitated, the therapist watches and waits and, in many cases, action will result naturally and spontaneously. And for Jane, that is exactly what happened. Jane, who had so much looked for instruction and guidance, began, unconsciously at first, to do things for herself, because they flowed automatically out of the inner shift. Thus, having confronted them in the photograph, she was able to make her family more aware of her own needs and to say what she wanted without fear or guilt.

Most importantly, we have seen how, as symbols of past trauma within her family, the photographs helped her to extricate herself from a tangled snare of self-condemnation and blame and to move into a recognition of her anger with others. She had been able to express her aggression through the photographs for the first time in her life, confronting the internalised persecutory aspects of herself. Her initial low energy, sapped by the strain of keeping strong feelings repressed, gave way to an increased vigour, as she was enabled to rid herself of old bitternesses and frustrations. Thus, in time, she could risk a more fulfilling life, because she was less afraid of failure.

Catharsis

Jane's experiences of using her photographs in an active way, especially towards the end of therapy, illustrate their power in the facilitation of catharsis. Catharsis refers to the discharge of emotion, and photographs have a definite function here because they stimulate strong, often repressed memories and feelings. In an accepting atmosphere, the patient will have an opportunity to release these emotions. Such a cathartic experience is not, however, enough in itself to promote real change; it enables inner pressures to come to the surface, so that therapist and patient can then explore their source and meaning.

Without the subsequent search for insight, the relief through catharsis may be transitory. One needs to reflect on the experience, to process it, to enquire and to wonder; indeed, wondering in itself has a large part to play in the therapeutic endeavour. Photographs are continually enticing us to wonder. Jane's cathartic experiences with photographs were accompanied with a search for meaning and a wondering that was largely initiated, at this stage in therapy, by Jane herself.

Here it will be seen that she was in control, taking responsibility for herself, leading the way. She used the photographs in a manner that enabled material from her unconscious to emerge, so that internalised persecutory figures could be 'killed off' and discarded. Thus, she was able to alter somewhat the relationship she had with these internal objects, to move towards ridding herself of the wholly damaging elements, through addressing their external representations in the photographs. Through the medium of the photographs, Jane could safely discharge hitherto repressed murderous feelings – to kill the image, without harming the real person at all.

The concrete evidential characteristics of the photograph, its solid and tangible quality and its firm physicality make it an especially good medium for such work in therapy, enabling people literally to get in touch with the images and to regress to earlier experiences. The preserved pictures from the past helped recreate and revivify past scenarios in the present and thus aided Jane's regression to earlier painful times. They permitted a reliving and a re-experiencing of the repressed pain. In order to help a patient through such an experience with photographs, the therapist needs to use the skills of immediacy, to stay with what is happening in the here and now, and to be able to reflect and respond in the moment.

Play

Through 'playing' with the images, Jane was actively able to create a longed-for situation with her parents, transforming the photographs to fit with her inner wishes. She well knew that this activity could not change the past, but such playing helped her more fully discover her own power in the present. In graphically transforming the past symbols of her helplessness, she was enabled to change inner defeating attitudes that had gripped her from childhood. She could lay the ghosts of powerlessness that had haunted her, robbing them of their control over her present self. In this way, myths about herself began to be shed; as the glimpses of her own strength increased, she was able to develop a fresh view of herself and the world and experience a 'change of consciousness' (Bonime 1962: 258).

Whilst Jane discovered some powerful and primitive feelings of hate towards members of her family, such play with photographs also revealed the tenderness that she felt. It facilitated, therefore, an awareness of ambivalence and the realisation that it is acceptable to have more than one set of feelings. We have seen in Chapter 2 how photographs hide meanings. Jane also saw how her pictures reflected opposite sets of feelings within the family because they could be seen on two levels: she perceived the smiles of the loving family, and also the depressed, angry, hating feelings underneath.

As Jane continued weekly to explore her photographs in therapy, we have seen how she became bolder and more daring in her use of them, risking the release of pent up emotions more overtly than before. This repeated perusal of the same photographs over many sessions represented a working through of difficult issues, especially those in relation to her father. As she returned to the same time-worn images, the same feelings would recur, yet on each occasion there was some small shift in attitude.

In addition, repeated looking at the powerful images seemed to soften them and, through this familiarity, Jane became more daring and courageous in utilising them. At this stage, photographs can profitably be combined with other therapeutic procedures. Techniques from psychodrama and Gestalt therapy, amongst many other approaches, may be beneficial in terms of the therapeutic use of photographs. Thus, feelings may be projected onto the pictures, as they are shouted at or cried over; faces can be changed, mouths gagged, eyes poked out, bodies dismembered and – perhaps – repaired. Figures can be moved or otherwise manoeuvred and controlled.

The patient may have been afraid to express any strong feelings in relationships, because of an unconscious fear of the power of such emotions. The photograph provides an opportunity for the expression of murderous feelings, of long repressed savage fantasies. Used in a therapeutic setting, it becomes a container within which such feelings and fantasies can be discharged safely.

Termination issues

Jane's gradual and symbolic taking back of the 'processed' photographs as therapy drew to a close helped her to separate from me. She had entrusted to me symbolic aspects of herself, and so the photographs had come to represent the strength of the therapeutic alliance. They were her personal and secret symbols, which she had risked sharing with me, so that we could jointly be creative with them. Thus they represented a bond between us, the memory of which Jane could hold inside her long after therapy had finished.

In addition, through internalising the elements of the therapy that would give her strength in the future, Jane felt ready to face the world with greater confidence. Her improved self-image meant that she could feel freer to 'play' in her life outside therapy, too. She took up golf, soon becoming proficient at it, enjoying the praise and attention she earned, and even daring to risk competitions. She began reading a little; she felt excited and validated by the fact that I actually wanted her permission to be *in* my book. Jane was also able to say a firm 'no' to the annual suggestion that she cook the Christmas meal for the whole extended family. She gained a clearer perception of own role in her difficulties, thus giving her control over them and creating a healthier sense of self.

There were, of course, areas of vulnerability remaining; she still found her sister's illness hauntingly difficult – and felt the old inferiority feelings at times. But she came to realise that her considerably deprived childhood meant that some residual problems would inevitably remain and she would have to accept this. Because of her emotionally impoverished past, she had had totally unrealistic expectations of what was 'normal' or reasonable in terms of feelings. She now realised that the end of therapy was not going to mean the end of all problems or that everything would be perfect; whilst she was disappointed and somewhat disillusioned at this, it did help her panic less about her own 'imperfections' and turn towards the aspects of herself and her life that had changed.

What Jane experienced as therapy neared its end was some disappointment that all would not be cured and solved in her life, that she would be left with some problems. The scars remained; I could neither erase them from her experience, nor from her pictures of the past – inner and outer; I was not the magical therapist for whom she had longed:

> The psychotherapy patient must also come to this heavy piece of understanding, that he does *not* need the therapist. The most important thing that each man must learn no one else can teach him. Once he accepts this disappointment, he will be able to stop depending on the therapist, the guru who turns out to be just another struggling human being. Illusions die hard, and it is painful to yield to the insight that a grown-up can be no man's disciple. This discovery does not mark the end of the search, but a new beginning.
>
> (Kopp 1980: 41)

> The Zen master warns 'If you meet Buddha on the road, kill him!' This admonition points up that no meaning that comes from outside ourselves is real. The Buddhahood of each of us has already been obtained.
>
> (Kopp 1980: 140)

As we have seen, Jane began to discover meanings from within herself, and it was after this that she moved towards termination in therapy. She had tried long and hard to work on separation from her sick sister; at an intellectual level, at least, she could now understand that she was entitled to live her own life, despite her sister's illness, in a way that, as a child, she could not separate from her father's psychiatric problems.

In contemplating the secret return of the photographs to her mother, Jane was symbolically shedding some of the damaging past experiences. Photographs are very valuable in helping people to mourn and end lost or destructive relationships in that they offer images of the past in the present for reassessment and the completion of unfinished business. The separation is inner as well as outer. Patients can be helped to finally take their leave of past figures that have been internalised and still feel powerful inside. In Chapter 7, there will be further examples of the use of photographs to help people through their grief and through the process of separation.

What Jane brought into therapy was a set of partial personal truths, an assortment of family myths, a scramble of memories screened by years of anxiety. Her self-image, sealed in the negativity of bitter experience, was distorted and garbled, parodied by fear, so that she did not know who she was. To find out, she had to journey inwards and backwards to take another look, to re-tell, to re-view her own life story. The photographs served as a visual *aide-mémoire* in this, helping her describe and reinterpret her experience, rectify omissions, restore true perspectives.

Chapter 5

A closer look at the family album
Searching for clues to the past

What novel – or what else in the world – can have the epic scope of a photograph album? May our Father in heaven, the untiring amateur who each Sunday snaps us from above, at an unfortunate angle that makes for hideous foreshortening, and pastes our pictures, properly exposed or not, in his album, guide me safely through this album of mine.

(Grass 1962: 49)

The previous chapters have described and illustrated the process of therapy and how photographs can fit into it. I shall now begin to take a closer look at the family album in a way that will continue the development of the therapist's skills in using and learning to 'read' photographs.

Once the secret language of photographs becomes understood, we may detect in them key clues to the past. As therapy progresses, these clues – silent, telling messages concealed behind the image – will come to reveal much about the nature of present interaction. The principal aim of this chapter is to prepare the ground for an understanding, through photographs, of such interactional patterns in therapy.

'THE FAMILY JEWELS'

The family album functions as a precious record, a unique chronicle of the family's life cycle and its history. It preserves ancestors long dead, revealing to subsequent generations aspects of their history; it shows them how their parents looked when they were young and documents their courtship, wedding and early marriage. It registers the birth of each child, the first day at school, sports days, graduations; it illustrates some of the changes that occur within the family as it grows and develops.

It is most often a prized possession, regarded as a treasure-chest of memories; one album was even entitled 'The Family Jewels'. Such a collection of photographs is an important signifier of a family's identity, an emblem of its singularity, its distinctiveness. It describes and delineates the family as a special group of people, set apart from the rest.

This immense significance of the family album to the patient makes it a most effective adjunct to individual, marital or family therapy. The therapist, therefore, needs to maintain an acute awareness of the centrality and symbolic meaning of the family album in her patients' lives, approaching it with an attitude of insightful care.

THE FAMILY ALBUM IN THERAPY

What is its contribution to the therapeutic process?

The family album assists the therapist in her assessment of patients; it can serve as a way to explain and illustrate personal, marital and family history to the therapist during the initial stages of therapy. Sometimes, photographs can be used as an additional tool in the making of genograms, contributing to the creation of a kind of visual family tree. This helps the therapist to gain a view of the relationships, the hierarchies, the culture, myths, norms and customs that make up the family system.

As the photographs are described, the patient's narrative will expand to include many peripheral details about the people in the pictures. The therapist will hear about the traditions, stereotypes and attitudes within the family and she will be given a sense of the chronology of family events and experiences. Both patients and therapist will gain a clear picture of the changes over the years in individuals and in the family as a whole, exploring the meaning of these changes for the family and the people within it.

Additionally, such photographs enable therapist and patients to observe how people are represented and to identify required 'camera behaviour'; they permit a study of family norms, its rules about style, expectations about dress, public conduct, presentation of self. They may also pinpoint alliances within the family and may help reveal family secrets and myths.

The pictures can also provide a basis for the telling of a family story, and an opportunity to describe the feelings and the reality behind poses and smiles. In marital or family work, memories can be checked out with others, and disagreements or inconsistencies in recollection can be challenged and discussed. Thus they encourage the beginning of dialogue and conversation within therapy, and a sharing of feelings about self and others.

The album also helps people to reconnect with family members who have died or are out of touch for other reasons. There is a reminder of forgotten relationships, forgotten lives. There is an opportunity to take another look at childhood, this time through the eyes of an adult, re-meeting the key figures in a past. People can revisit the past together, and face feelings that may have been left without resolution. Questions are posed, memories triggered, both shared and individual; there is review, reflection, a looking back, a tracing of family patterns of behaviour.

And, finally, the photographs will provide a base from which patients can begin to reframe their lives, bring about a transformation, take a fresh look at the self in the world. This involves the shedding of many preconceptions, assumptions and myths, and a confrontation with internal resistances to change.

Laying the foundation: learning to 'read' the family photograph

Family photographs may be brought into therapy in many ways: in shoe-boxes, plastic bags, biscuit tins, neat albums, or even in large suitcases. The term 'family album', as used here, will, therefore, apply to any of these collections of photographs, in whatever manner they are presented.

What does the therapist endeavour to help the patient look for in the family album? How does this kind of looking differ from the usual study of such photographs?

It differs in that photographs are 'read', with an analytic attitude, a new way of seeing. The therapist will at first feel into the photograph, sensing the overall atmosphere and the emotions in the family group. She will notice and question the way in which the people have grouped themselves and will also look at the setting, the background and the objects in the picture. As she does so, there will be a careful, sensitive checking out with the patient, so that the focus of therapy is not deflected by the therapist's own assumptions.

When exploring a family album with patients, it is important to become aware of moods and expressions, actions and gestures within the photographs. What does all this mean? Observe the positions and postures and determine whether these give information about the family hierarchies, its customs and cultures.

Try, if possible, to discover who assembled the album and what thoughts and feelings were experienced during its compilation. Are there patterns, conscious or unconscious, that emerge in the way the album has been put together? What is seen as the purpose of the family album? What was the motivation behind the taking and assembling of the pictures?

We have seen how photographs encourage us to ask questions; as we peruse the family album, its powerful impact will produce a host more. Some answers may be unavailable, lost in time; others may help elucidate and clarify.

We may wonder: who took the photographs? Of whom are they taken? Who possesses the family album? How frequently is it perused and by whom? When are the photos taken and of what?

We will attempt to understand what all this information tells us about the way in which the family organises itself and interacts. We will notice whether there are many photographs, or very few. Does a lack of photographs reflect a family that was uninterested in itself and its children, or is it an indication of financial hardship? Conversely, do large quantities of pictures reflect pleasure and pride or obsessiveness and control?

Try to observe whether there are aspects in the album that were missed on first perusal, and which have only become evident on a more detailed study of the pictures. Do the pictures change after you have heard the narrative or studied them in more depth? Do they appear different now?

As a therapist, it is important to notice how the people are relating to each other, physically and emotionally. It will be noted whether there are indications of equality between the adults in the picture, or signs of dominance and passivity. Where there are couples, the therapist will consider whether one partner appears to be more attentive and loving than the other. She will help her patients to detect patterns, repeated examples of similar scenarios.

The importance of a series of photographs

In beginning the search for these patterns within the family, it is most important to remember that a collection of photographs is needed if repeated gestures and interactions are to be discovered. If a certain kind of positioning is apparent in only one photograph, there may be some doubt as to its validity as an indicator of some deeper meaning; chance obviously plays a part in the capturing of an uncharacteristic expression or position.

A solitary photograph captures only a single instant and this may – or may not – be an instant that typifies many others. Only if the accompanying narrative confirms that this captured moment is reflective of the whole picture, can real attention be given to the message of the single photograph.

Patrick Lichfield highlights the reductionist aspect of photography that may lead to all sorts of erroneous assumptions – sometimes rather dangerous ones:

> If you press the button at precisely the same moment as the doorbell rings, you will produce a portrait of someone who always looks a little distracted. If you manage to capture a fleeting moment of indigestion, the subject will always appear bad-tempered. And if you trap a genuine smile, he or she will always seem to be the nicest person in the world. Clothes and props also assume a larger-than-life importance. (Show a happily married mother of five with a wine bottle in her hand and she will be branded for life as an inveterate alcoholic; picture a normally pin-striped businessman in his gardening clothes and he will be transformed into a down-and-out.)
> (Lichfield 1981: 158)

Therefore, in order to trace repeated family patterns, a collection of photographs is preferable. The focus will be on looking for recurring styles of relating and processes of interaction that trace through time. Viewed within the context of a verbal description, these may provide visual evidence of conflicts and alliances within the family. If there is not a series of pictures, however, it is still possible for the patient's accompanying narrative to confirm whether the camera has recorded a fragment of a fixed pattern or if it has merely snatched an untypical moment.

Looking at proximity

Whilst analysing family patterns, take account of the space between the people in the photographs, for this may give clues as to whether the family is enmeshed and over-close in its way of interacting, or distanced and emotionally cut off from one other. Many family snaps show people with their arms folded, behind their backs, or with their hands sunk deep within their pockets – anything to avoid physical contact with other family members. Consideration should be given to such detail as an absence of warm expression, or whether the feeling of the photograph is loving and close. Perhaps, on the other hand, there is a claustrophobic atmosphere. These details may say much about the family's way of being.

Marion felt that her mother had always favoured her brother. On all the family photographs, mother was holding Daniel close to her, whilst Marion was trailing some distance behind, or sitting apart. In therapy, Marion decided to experiment with her pictures. She brought photocopies of them, so she would not have to destroy them, and also so that she could try various ways of playing with the same photographs. She cut out the figures and began to rearrange the pictures according to her wishes and longings. Eventually, she deftly managed to place herself in her mother's arms, and to put her brother on the ground beside her. She was only able to do this, however, after she had worked on her self-image in therapy. Up to then, she had felt that she had 'no right' to be held by mother, for she did not deserve such nurturing.

'This photograph says it all'

Look at Photograph 13. It belongs to the child on the right of the picture, Jeffrey, now an adult. What can you see? Can you attempt to 'read' this photograph? At first, this may look like an ordinary family snapshot, one of the many that lie in the countless albums, each seemingly resembling the other. But look closer. The photograph contains the story of a family, and within it are the subtle clues to individual and family issues of considerable import and significance.

See how the father is holding the little girl close to him, leaving no space between them, and how she in turn holds his arm, leaning against him contentedly. Look at the young child on his other arm; notice the distance here, between the man and his child, who sits uncomfortably on his father's

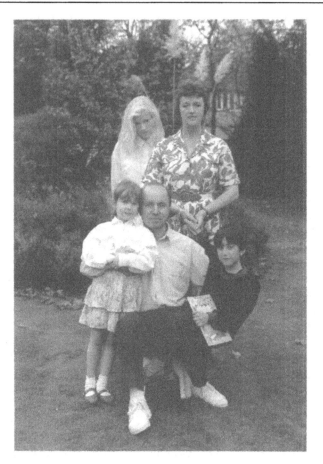

Photograph 13
Posed by models

knee. Unlike the close physical contact with his daughter, the father holds the boy almost at arm's length – one can see the mother's dress behind, through the gap his arm makes. The boy reaches awkwardly behind his father's head to grasp his mother's hands – perhaps for security? Beside the woman, the older girl, who is touching no one, but standing slightly behind mother, looks wary and shy, vulnerable, perhaps angry. She is a little outside the family, somehow. Jeffrey feels that she looks lost – does her position express this?

We may also wonder at the positions of the parents in the photograph. Father is sitting at mother's feet; this is quite rare in family pictures, for most often, it is the woman who sits, and the man who stands behind. The woman does not touch her husband, who has his back to her. She seems almost to be the dominant figure in the picture.

Jeffrey relates how he was 'a bit of a mother's boy – and I clung to her', because he felt she was more understanding to him than his father was. He comments on the fact that he is holding a book:

> This feels like something to hold onto, like a prop. It reminds me now that I was very closed emotionally. I was giving myself something to do, a way to close up, and also to cling on. It isn't an open position, it is tight and tense – that is how I felt a lot of the time. This photograph says it all. It is exactly how it looks. Without any explanation, it is possible to see how the physical positions totally reflect every aspect of the emotional states and relationships in my family.

Here is an example of a photograph that serves as the kind of hologram referred to in Chapter 3. Jeffrey's photograph, although only in itself a small part of his whole collection, mirrors many of his others, and represents aspects of the family's history and interaction. It is astonishingly reflective of wider issues, summing up several of the themes in its owner's life history.

Reading between the photographs: significant omissions

In some albums, there may be significant omissions; whilst there needs to be attention given to the people who feature most or least in a family album, it is equally important to enquire about any such absences. Our photograph albums may contain many gaps, but these are usually noticed only by those who have inside knowledge of the family history. We have seen in Chapter 4 how Jane's wedding album painfully revealed to her the gaps left by her sick father's absence; such omissions, in the context of a personal narrative, may be heavily laden with meaning, signalling issues of considerable import.

For instance, whilst exploring her family pictures, Maggie came across a seaside picture that had unconsciously made a telling statement about a family situation through its omissions. She soon discovered that many of her pictures symbolically expressed aspects of what was happening in her family.

Maggie is a photographer and artist from Australia, and she had brought her family over to London for a year while she did further training. During my research for this book, I placed an advertisement in a journal for people to get in touch if they had photographs that they wished to explore in a therapeutic way. Maggie replied, and we arranged for her to spend the weekend with me, so that we could explore her pictures together. Maggie wanted to learn about photo-therapy, so our relationship was mutually productive.

Maggie enigmatically titled Photograph 14 'Empty-headed parents'; this unconsciously symbolised an ongoing family issue. The seaside photograph

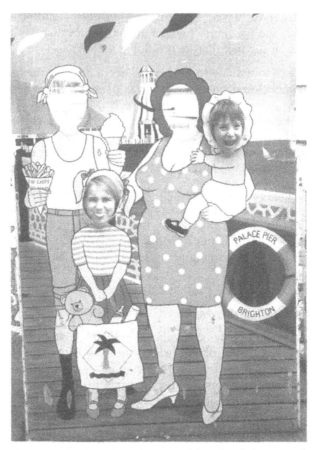

Photograph 14
© Maggie Wilson

shows Maggie's children with their heads through the cut out picture-board – but there are empty spaces for the parents, and the beach is visible behind. Aesthetically, Maggie finds this pleasingly surrealistic in tone. She feels the photograph is representative of an ongoing family theme, which concerns the absence of parent figures. Her partner is working hard and is not able to be with the children very often. Maggie herself is busy with her studies. She feels that the beach photograph signifies the lack of parental presence in the family at this time.

Maggie asks: 'Have I unconsciously exposed my children's reality though the camera, whilst my partner and I busily get on with our lives?' (Wilson 1991: 27).

Sometimes, there are noticeable gaps in an album, left by the absent few; such gaps may have much significance in terms of the family.

Frequently, it is the people who have the same role in the family who are missing from photographs across the generations. Rachel, whose father died when she was very young, was herself now divorced. She showed me the family photographs, where two generations of women were pictured with their children. Each family was lacking a father. She felt sad that this pattern has been repeated.

Many such omissions may yield important information about the family history, its culture and its attitudes. Jonathan figured prominently in his family's photograph album from its beginning; then, suddenly, it seemed, he was banished from its pages. This abrupt exclusion reflected a rift between Jonathan and his parents that persists to this day, for he married a woman of a different religion, and that was unacceptable to his family.

In most family albums, there are periods of time when no photographs are taken. Usually this is during illness, separation or crisis. An exploration of a patient's family album, with an eye to such time-gaps, may help reveal and pinpoint traumatic phases in a family's life.

A TESTIMONY FROM THE PAST: DISCOVERING THE MESSAGES BEHIND THE IMAGE

How can the therapist use the information gleaned from this new way of looking at the family album? By what methods can she enable patients to let the pictures speak, helping people to interpret their coded visual signals, to translate their secret language? How can she use such pictures therapeutically, to understand the clues about the family's systems, its network of relationships and its unconsciously repeated patterns?

Now that therapist and patient have begun to 'read' photographs, the once lifeless images become activated, releasing floods of recollections and communications. Once these basic 'reading' skills have been mastered, questions are asked, patterns are identified, memories return. Messages from important figures in the patient's past are recalled and these help the therapist to build up a significant picture of the patient's early life experiences.

The photograph album will mirror back these communications from the past for analysis and instruction and it is most important to be able to identify and pinpoint such messages with patients in therapy, for they can symbolically encapsulate a parent's attitude towards the child and thus may be seen as having influenced patients and shaped their being, contributing to adult patterns of interaction.

In the next chapter, I shall move to an exploration of these patterns of interaction within marriage and family. But before such a detailed examination, the roots of these patterns must be unearthed, for they lie deeply embedded in the past. There follows a selection of ways in which photographs can afford us vital assistance in tracing the development of such multigenerational forms of family interaction.

Patterns of health

Powerful responses from the significant figures in the patient's life are communicated in a variety of ways; the photograph records them and shows, sometimes quite graphically, how the child was treated within the family. It permits the therapist to feel strongly the atmosphere in which the patient has grown up, and thus to learn to understand at a deeper level.

Photographs will reveal not only the negative communications, but also the positive and empathic responses which patients have experienced, and will bequeath to their children: ways of being that will be nurturing and sustaining, for patterns of interaction do not die with people. Through the photographs and the contrasts that they present, the patient can be helped to differentiate strengthening parental responses from the more negative ones.

These healthy strands can be traced, gratifyingly, and with some joy, through the majority of family albums that are brought into therapy; it is important to help the patient discover these as well as the less positive ones, to see how the photograph confirms such patterns, for it, too, does not die with the people it portrays. Such positive communications to children form the basis of their self-image, and their ability to love and relate in later life. The photograph will, therefore, testify to the warmth, caring and love that has been expressed within the family (see Photograph 15).

Holding

Frequently, evidence of how safe and secure children feel in the arms of an adult is to be gleaned from their demeanour and expressions. We may learn from their family albums how patients reacted to being held, and how they hold their own children. This will help us to understand their often unremembered early experience, and to see how this may have coloured subsequent patterns of relating to others.

The eminent psychoanalyst, Heinz Kohut, makes such use of a patient's family photograph album to aid in the process of assessment and diagnosis, and to provide a kind of evidence about his patient's childhood:

There was every indication, both from external evidence and from the over-all flavour of Mr Z's personality, that the unremembered earliest part of his life, perhaps the first year or year and a half, had been a happy one. However severely distorted the personality of his mother basically might have been, as will be discussed later on, she was quite young when the patient was born, and the intense relationship with her baby might, as long as he was still small and the interweaving of her with him still phase-appropriate, have brought out her healthiest attitudes. At any rate, to all appearances, he was the apple of her eye,

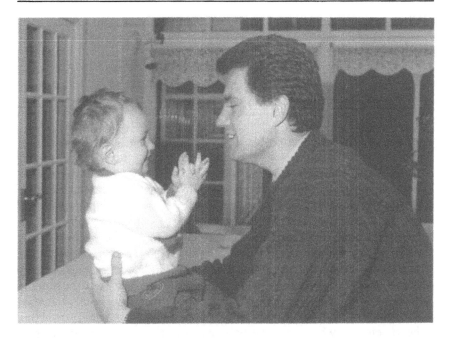

Photograph 15

and the father, too, seems to have been pleased with him – at least as far as could be judged from entries in a baby book and snapshots and home movies that had been taken by the young couple. Whether his picture was taken as he was held by his mother, or, occasionally, by the father, his facial expression and general demeanour seemed that of a happy, healthy baby.

(Kohut 1979: 4)

The way in which children are held is extremely important in developing their ability to relate to others and to grow into healthy adults. Touch is a basic human need, and its absence may create difficulties in relationships in later life. If children are held – physically and emotionally – with real affection, they will carry loved and loving feelings with them into adulthood. If they are not, they experience an inner emptiness and a desperate longing that remains with them, creating difficulties that will pervade their adult relationships and their own abilities to parent.

Such adults may find their way into therapy, where they will hopefully experience a sense of being securely held through the emotional containment and support that the therapist can offer. Whilst the therapist will be unable to compensate for the patient's childhood lack, the hope is that she will be able to give the patient a new experience of secure, non-possessive care. The patient needs to be seen, heard and contained in a way that feels confirming and safe. Then he or she will feel secure enough to relax into the process of therapy without fear of being 'dropped' or roughly handled, in emotional terms.

Winnicott emphasised the importance of the child being held in a containing way, if he or she is to grow into a healthy adult. He explains that holding helps the baby to relax and regress into a state of 'unintegration', describing a stage

> . . . in which a well-cared-for developing baby can relax and uninte-grate, and tolerate (but only just tolerate) feeling 'mad' in the uninte-grated state. Then a stage forward is made, a step towards independence, and a loss forever of the capacity to be unintegrated except in madness or in the specialised conditions provided in psychotherapy. After this the word is disintegration.

> . . . it can be said that where the holding of a baby is perfect (and it often is, since mothers know just how to do it) then the baby can get confidence even in the live relationship, and can unintegrate while being held. This is the richest type of experience. Often, however, the holding is variable or even spoiled by anxiety (mother's over-control against dropping) or by anxiousness (mother's trembling, hot skin, over-acting heart, etc.) in which case the baby cannot afford to relax. Relaxation then only comes with exhaustion.

> (Winnicott 1991: 118–19)

Within the photograph album, there are many photographs which show children being carried, cradled, touched, held. Some parents demonstrate a containing and secure way of holding; some reveal a care-less style, seemingly unaware of the child, clasping him or her limply and unsafely. Others show the kind of anxious, over-firm holding of which Winnicott speaks. It is interesting to note how graphically a collection of photographs can indicate the absence or presence of holding, and also its nature and quality.

Listening

It may be surprising to consider the fact that, as well as revealing whether people have been seen and held adequately as children, the photograph can 'tell' us whether they have been *heard*.

Iris brought a photograph of her children sitting with her father (Photograph 16). Here, he is reading to his grandchildren, but they are obviously not the slightest bit impressed with his story; they are, in fact, watching television. But grandfather continues to read, oblivious of their inattention.

Iris reflects that this photograph reminds her of her own childhood, symbolically. Father was always out at work, and when he was with his children, he never seemed to listen to them. Iris adds:

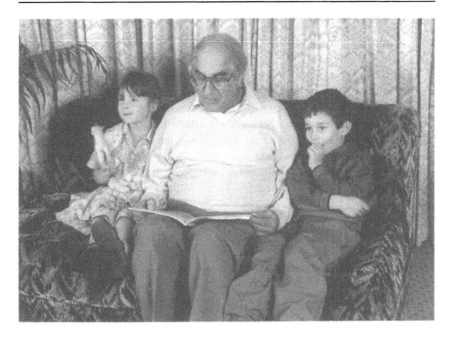

Photograph 16
Posed by models

> I am very aware of the necessity of listening to children now. I can't bear it when people don't listen to them. I have joined an organisation that helps parents to listen, because this issue has become so important to me.

Iris had never before realised how powerfully this photograph symbolised important aspects of her own childhood. She was also relieved to discover a photograph of herself in the album where she is quite obviously listening lovingly and attentively to her child, who is reading aloud to her.

Learning

Additionally, the photograph may reveal how children learn through emulating their parents, absorbing aspects of adult behaviour as they develop their own unique identity. It can show whether they are tense and anxious within their family – or relaxed and at ease, unconsciously mimicking parental body-language and expression. A relaxed identification with parents reveals the presence of trust, a most important element in a child's development. If children feel able to trust their parents, they will be able to learn from and imitate them. They will also be able to trust themselves and others in adult relationships.

Sibling relationships and birth order

Within the family albums brought to therapy, there are many childhood scenes of patients with their siblings; through them, the therapist may glean many important details about the nature of such relationships, for experiences with siblings will have an influence on adult ways of relating.

Gerald brought several photographs of himself, his parents and his siblings. He had problems in his present life with closeness and intimacy, both on a physical and emotional level. He was having difficulty relating this to past experience and was heavily denying any links. Towards the end of a rather blank and withdrawn therapy hour, Gerald turned to gaze at a photograph of himself and his three siblings and suddenly began to sob in a desperate way.

When he had recovered a little, he was able to share that, for the first time ever, he had seen that nobody was touching anyone else in the photograph; everyone was physically separate. This realisation – that at an unconscious level his family was showing how difficult were closeness and intimacy – released a flood of painful memories of isolation in the cold house of his childhood. He was able, after this, to get in touch with more feelings that had long been repressed and to begin to understand the roots of his marital difficulties in the present.

Whilst looking in therapy at a photograph of herself and her brother as children, Beverley remembered that she had been forced to rest her head on her brother's shoulder. Until we looked closely at the picture, she had not noticed a small detail in the lower left corner. This was a smudged image of her mother's hand, which, in the seconds before the picture had been taken, was pressing Beverley's head down. The camera had caught the withdrawing hand for posterity. It had frozen an instant that symbolised Beverley's deep feelings of being secondary to others in her family in terms of feelings and needs. As an adult, Beverley had a great fear of any relationship, including the therapy one with me, feeling that her needs could never be met and that she was unlovable. The photograph, with its 'mistake', was a symbol of the childhood origin of these problems and signified the main issues in the relationship between herself, her parents and her brother.

We will inevitably encounter in our patients' albums photographs of sisters and brothers interacting, perhaps playing together, or posing for a parent's camera. We may detect there the pain of envy and rivalry, the distress of feeling displaced by a 'new arrival', the enormous gap when a sibling dies, the joy of companionship, the love and the hate that become a significant part of the patchwork of formative relationships in a person's life.

Beth showed me a picture of herself and two sisters standing with their nanny, who holds the youngest in her arms. The small child on the left of the picture is crying and, at first glance, it is not apparent exactly why,

However, on taking a closer look at the photograph, the reason becomes clear. The child in her nanny's arms has her foot dangling dangerously near her sister's head, and she looks rather self-satisfied. Once this quite subtle detail is spotted, it is obvious what has occurred seconds before the camera clicked. The kick symbolised a pattern of surreptitious sibling rivalry that continued within this family throughout childhood.

Birth order and the resulting roles and positions in the family can have considerable influence on the development of the child and on the nature of adult relationships. Such roles are often replicated within a marital relationship, and may be detected in the transference with the therapist. Thus, an eldest child, who may have always had a looking-after role in the family, may perpetuate this in marriage, and may also attempt to take charge of the therapy and the therapist.

It is interesting to note how these roles and positions are reflected in the photograph, and how strong are the feelings associated with recognising one's designated family place. Peter, a middle child, noticed, to his chagrin, how he was always in between his siblings on their family photographs; he felt this symbolised a sense of himself as a 'middling' sort of person, never excelling at anything. Within his marital relationship, the pattern had been repeated; he felt a sort of unnecessary encumbrance in the family, just as he had felt as a child.

This middle position on a photograph is a different kind of position from the child who is the focus of attention. Even though both may be in the middle, the latter feels central rather than 'middling'. Sometimes a new baby becomes the photographic centre of attraction; this positioning often represents the change in family dynamics that is inevitably brought about by the arrival of a new sibling.

It may also be apparent that some families favour boys or girls, with the favoured sex occupying prime positions, on a parent's knee, for example, whilst the other children appear less important in terms of positioning.

Socialisation

By means of a process of socialisation, the family has moulded its children to fit in with its norms and rules. In assembling the family album, further selection will ensure that these are preserved for posterity:

> Are there any rules about how people have to be in order to be included in your album? If so, those rules will probably mirror the rules about what people have to do to be loved in your family. Inclusion in the family album is a metaphor for inclusion in the family.
>
> (Weiser 1990: 115)

Jenny and Eric came together for marital therapy; their childhood photographs vividly reflected the socialisation that lay at the core of their current marital problems. Both partners were trapped in needing to please – or to rebel against – internalised critical parent figures, which constantly replayed messages to them from the past.

In turn, neither could feel good enough for the other, and each made impossible demands on their spouse. Eric's family photograph album showed how he had been the recipient of parental expectations of perfection, for he was rigidly posed, told to stand in certain ways that looked uncomfortable and difficult. These poses, he felt, reflected the unyielding and insensitive kind of parenting he had experienced. Yet, in the same way, he began to see that he was also expecting Jenny to fit in with the rigid ideas of his family and to be a 'perfectly posed' wife.

Jenny's pictures revealed a child with hair ostentatiously wound into tight, beribboned ringlets. But Jenny had very, very straight hair. She had endured the discomfort of having it regularly and painfully curled, very much against her will, for she loved to wear her hair straight and shiny.

However, Jenny, too, wanted her husband to fit into her image of how a husband should be. She veered between feeling consumed with guilt at not being as Eric wanted her, exhausting herself in her efforts to please him and, at the other extreme, rebelling against him and all that he stood for.

Both partners struggled with their own internal fears about not conforming to another's design for them, and worked to free their inner child from the stultifying rules of the past, which they had seen mirrored most powerfully in their photographs. Further, through the medium of these snapshots of the other's past, they saw the shared experiences they had had, and how they were repeating and perpetuating these within the marriage, to drastic effect.

'The look'

Children learn how to 'be' through parental instruction and they will learn what is desirable and what is unacceptable through cues from parents, both verbal and non-verbal. One most powerful way of communicating to children is through 'the look'. How often does one hear the statement: 'Father didn't have to tell me off, he just gave me one of his looks and I felt about two inches high. . . .'

The camera may have immortalised a specific parental look, a powerful gaze that has remained imprinted in the patient's mind, even long after the death of that parent. There may be captured someone's 'typical' expression, one that characterises a person, and his or her way of relating to others. The photograph will help patients think about the looks that they have reserved for their children. Are they generally approving and kind, or critical and judgemental? Will these looks be remembered with affection and fondness – or with resentment and hatred? Some looks bring comfort, others create fear; they speak silent volumes, and are often repeated constantly, to powerful effect.

Esther showed me her wedding photograph, where everybody was looking at the camera, except Esther's mother, who gazed at her daughter, smiling in a sort of indulgent way. Esther's explanation shows that this look has specific meaning for her in the whole context of her relationship with her mother:

> This look of mother's makes me cringe . . . I have seen it so often that I shudder at it, because it is a social look that says to the world 'This is my daughter', as if we are really so close. But the truth is that we aren't close, and this is just a public veneer. It is often the look that she gives me on photographs.

Derek has a picture of his dead mother which he takes out from time to time, especially when he needs comfort. Her eyes are soft and warm, and her look is one that gave Derek much consolation and hope from babyhood. Now that she is gone, her special look is preserved in his memory, and the feelings are reaffirmed by the picture.

Photographs can also indicate an absence of looks, a lack of attention; Jacky brought me a photograph that expressed her feelings about her father's inattentiveness; mother was playing happily with her children, whilst father sat engrossed in his book. She saw this as representative of her experience of him as totally uninvolved with his children, leaving mother to do all the playing.

REFLECTIONS OF PAST MESSAGES IN THE PRESENT

I have focused on the way in which photographs may be 'read' in therapy with a view to recognising photographic clues to early experience.

As we now move on through the family album in therapy, we will see further how these past messages have influenced the present, for similar responses repeat themselves through its pages. Multigenerational modes of relating fix the past in the present and often create trauma and distress for those who inherit them.

The family album can reveal, to those who will look, such recurring patterns of circular, futile behaviour that may have existed for decades. They show how, blinkered by fear, unconscious of inner motivations, people retrace together the same patterns of behaviour over time.

When couples and families come into therapy, they are most often trapped and caught within the complex weave of their shared pathology. At some level, however, in seeking help, they are wanting to discard the legacy of distress that has been passed on through many lifetimes and to alter the destructive images of the past.

Chapter 6

The search continues
Exploring images of interaction

Photography makes us aware for the first time of the optical unconscious, just as psychoanalysis discloses the instinctual unconscious.

(Benjamin 1972: 7)

I shall now proceed to an examination of the family album in the light of theories of marital and family interaction. In this chapter, there will be examples of how photographs can be used in therapy to facilitate patients' understanding of these interactional patterns and of the self in relationships. The individual will be helped to gain an awareness of self within the family system, and the role that he or she plays out within that system.

Photographs may also reveal how differentiated or enmeshed in age-old systems are the individuals within the family. As the album is worked through in the therapy situation, individuals, couples and families may be enabled to identify and recognise the network of patterns in which they have become trapped. We have begun to see how these interactions become even more constricting if they are allowed to continue unhampered by consciousness.

In addition, as therapy deepens, the photographs, with their unique ability to provide a passageway into the unconscious, allow patients to get in touch with hidden and repressed feelings; the case of Klaus and Louise will vividly illustrate this.

Building on the information from Chapter 5, we shall see how the photograph can inform us about the way in which early parental messages influence subsequent relationships. Issues introduced in the previous chapter will therefore now be extended into a wider exploration of how the family album can be used to identify interactional rhythms and themes, charting their transmission through the generations. For where there are family groups, such patterns will tend to intensify and proliferate; these will inevitably be illustrated in the photograph.

REFLECTIONS OF SELF IN THE OTHER: THE PHOTOGRAPH AND MARITAL INTERACTION

There follows an example of the way in which photographs can be used to considerable effect in marital therapy. This will lead on to an explanation of aspects of psychoanalytic theories of marital interaction; an understanding of such theories is essential if photographs are to be used with couples in therapy.

A picture of a marriage – Klaus and Louise

The kind of parental looks and messages that are illustrated in the family album of Klaus, whom we first met in Chapter 3, reveal the origins of his difficulty with relationships as an adult. They also help illustrate how the nature of childhood experiences will directly influence subsequent marital and family interaction.

Klaus first came into therapy alone. He was emotional, guilty and depressed about the relationship with his wife and child. He portrayed himself as the black sheep of his family, critical of those around him. His wife, Louise, was desperately unhappy at the treatment she received from her husband, whom she experienced as abusive and aggressive. It was only afterwards that he appeared to reflect on the damage he had done.

Klaus described how as a child he had been treated in this abusive manner by his mother, always feeling blamed and bad. In his family album, he showed me some early photographs of himself with his mother. He saw that he looked uncomfortable, and that mother appeared to be hardly aware of her son, for she was endlessly posing, staring dreamily into space. She never seemed to be looking at him; there was an absence of warm and confirming looks from mother to child. Klaus felt that the pictures had nothing to do with him or his identity, but that he was used as a vehicle for his mother's needs, both in these pictures, and in his childhood in general. These pictures also confirmed to Klaus how his needs were not *heard*.

From the way Klaus presented his marital problems, it seemed as if he were expressing all the 'negative' feelings in the relationship; both he and his wife had labelled him as the one to blame, just as he had been labelled as a child. As the focus of our initial sessions seemed to be on difficulties in the marriage, it seemed important to suggest that Klaus's wife, Louise, be invited into therapy, so that we could begin to see the whole picture of the relationship.

Louise was willing to attend, but seemed from the beginning to be rather remote and to collude with the idea that it was Klaus who had the problems. On the surface, it appeared as if Louise was the 'good one', who never got angry, and stoically suffered her husband's moods. The couple were very polarised: Louise's apparent calm reasonableness contrasted with her husband's impulsive anger.

Yet, as Louise described her past, it became apparent that there were considerable similarities in the couple's childhood experiences, in that both had had distant or unavailable fathers, and mothers who were experienced as unloving and inattentive. As therapy progressed, it emerged that Louise had repressed much of her own rage and anger and had hidden it behind a protective screen of rationality. Klaus was therefore carrying a 'double dose' of anger for both partners.

Louise had never felt heard or valued as a child, and her mother was always busy looking after others. But there was no permission in her family to express feelings and, therefore, unconsciously, she chose a partner who could do this for her. She was projecting the anger and depressed feelings that she felt about her past and present situations onto her husband, and denying such feelings within herself.

It was a photograph of Klaus as a child that eventually allowed Louise to get in touch with and take responsibility for her own childhood feelings, which up to then had been difficult to express. Both seemed to find it hard to remember aspects of the past and I had wondered if they had any photographs. Louise had none, but Klaus brought an early family album to the following session. As he turned the pages, tears welled up in his eyes. He stopped at one particular picture (Photograph 17) and cried softly, staring at it for a long time. Louise sat beside him, absorbed, attentive, silent.

He began to speak:

'This was taken by my mother, soon after we arrived in Britain. (To me . . .) She had married an Englishman, you see.' I nodded. There was a long pause.

I said: 'It looks like there might be many feelings going on inside you, in that picture. . . .'

He responded quickly, desperately: 'I was miserable . . . and lonely, terribly lonely in a strange land. I felt . . . I felt like I feel now, sometimes . . . er . . . not contained, nobody to hold me, touch me . . . a sort of sensory deprivation, you know, empty, as if in the middle of a vessel, suspended, groping for the sides.'

He was crying. As usual, the focus, as far as problems were concerned, was on Klaus, who had unconsciously volunteered to be the designated patient. This fitted in with his life 'script' and allowed Louise to be 'free' of emotion.

She had been sitting, motionless, staring pensively at the photographs of her husband's sad childhood. At this point, though, she shuffled in her chair, *changing position*.

And then I noticed that, for the first time, she too was crying. She

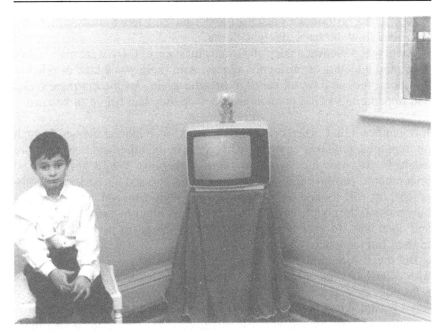

Photograph 17
Posed by a model

reached for a tissue and covered her face. We waited. I said softly, looking at Louise: 'This is touching both of you. . . .'

They continued to weep, together, for their separate, yet shared, childhood pain.

But Louise said through her tears: 'I am crying for Klaus's childhood . . . I can see the anxiety, the desperation in that picture. I am crying for all that *he* didn't have. . . .'

I knew that this was a moment to begin to help her to explore her own inner pain, to attempt to balance the interaction between them. I risked: 'Perhaps this resonates with some of your *own* early feelings. . . .'

She hesitated, uncomfortable at what must have felt like a confrontation from me. It was a tense moment, seemingly eternal, for she could have taken refuge in denial, leaving him still with the problems. Klaus turned his head to look towards her now, his gaze intense, supportive. Something in the room had already changed in this very small movement; for this was a moment when *his* problems were not the main focus.

Uneasily, warily she ventured into the new territory: 'I think I am . . . crying about the loneliness and feelings of unimportance *I* had as a child. . . . In that photograph of Klaus . . . I can see myself . . . unseen. . . .'

She was crying freely now.

'. . . I had no father's presence, and I haven't felt Klaus's either . . . and, somehow, he feels lonely with me.'

There was a silence, a deep and mournful silence; there were many more tears, and a feeling of profound sadness. And there was a kind of relief in the room, too, as if we all dared to breathe again, for the marriage scales had tipped and swayed precariously, before they had begun to balance.

It is significant that, when one spouse reflects on childhood themes through photographs, similar issues may be triggered in the other and become more available for conscious work in marital therapy. Whilst the husband remembered painful childhood traumas as he perused his personal photographs, his wife looked on, weeping for her own damaged inner child. As time passed, the couple began to relate to each other in a much more clear and open way, to understand each other's feelings, to be more balanced in their interaction.

But there were limitations to my therapeutic endeavour. Therapy ended with Klaus coming alone again which, in retrospect, was certainly a reflection of – and a collusion with – the marital system. As a couple, there was a partial avoidance of facing the depression about past losses, and the pain that this engendered as it was recreated in the marriage. Whilst there was much insight and understanding, and considerable change in the marital and family systems, ultimately some of these deeper issues remained largely unaffected by therapy. With an acceptance of these limitations, it seems important to reflect on how the photographs *did* aid any changes that were able to be made.

Even though Louise had no photographs of her own, and few conscious memories of her past, she became stimulated by her husband's sombre pictures, and was able to follow his lead and search within herself for internal images of her past. Klaus, in divulging and sharing feelings, helped towards freeing his partner. It is often the partner designated as the problem who eventually enables the other to become more in touch with feelings.

Louise recollected then that she had been trapped in an inherited family view of men as at fault and women as long-suffering victims; she also remembered that emotions were unacceptable in her family. For most of her childhood, she had felt unheard and unimportant.

As she became more aware of these patterns, she began to alter them. She expressed her feelings more assertively, became more immediate, less distant, and Klaus in turn was more able to get in touch with the nurturing and gentle side of himself that previously only Louise had expressed. He felt less need to scare her and his daughter, as his mother had scared him. Klaus and Louise were able to see more of the inner child in self and other, and to understand that, deep inside, both felt bad, unimportant, blameworthy. Klaus was able to see another part of his wife, a more vulnerable self, and thus to be less intolerant and punitive of her needs.

It would seem to me that one of the main sticking points in marriage occurs when neither spouse can see the child in the other, experiencing the other only as aggressive and irritating rather than needy and sad. Once they can see the child aspect, and the links to past experience, the present interaction tends to become less fraught. Using photographs in this way helps couples, literally, to see clearly the child in themselves and each other, to regress to a time before the cement of adult defences had begun to set firm.

As they bring the past into the present, photographs present patients undisputably with their childhood feelings – images of little faces etched with emotion. Then there will be an awareness of how, over the years, adults have learnt to conceal and pretend. Confronted with this cover-up in the presence of one's spouse in therapy, it is difficult to continue such pretence; very often it is then that defences are lowered.

The therapy with Klaus and Louise also illustrates the fact that the personal issues of one spouse in marital therapy will very often resonate with those of the other, so that, whilst it may appear that only one partner is the focus, in fact mutual issues are addressed. Self-discovery through the other and within the marriage is thus possible, and such photographs serve to aid this important process.

Psychoanalytic theories of marital interaction

The case of Klaus and Louise may be used to explain something of the process of marital therapy and to show how photographs may be used to confirm and understand aspects of unconscious interaction in marriage.

Selection of partner

Couples choose each other for many reasons – social, cultural and physical. At an unconscious level, however, they are attracted to each other because they share a similar problem, they are stuck at a corresponding stage in their emotional development and unconsciously recognise the same un-resolved needs in the other.

Such unmet needs from early life will be reawakened in marriage, in an unconscious attempt to use the opportunity to work through the problems associated with them. The hope is that each partner has chosen the other in order to recreate the shared past problems and thus work through them – for one cannot work through a problem without going into it again. But, in this way, marriage can also mean that the partners become desperately trapped in the problems once more.

Whilst the adult may consciously want to begin anew in a marital relationship, there are powerful unconscious bonds with important figures from the past that will influence the choice of spouse. So, Klaus and Louise chose a partner who could recreate with them the similar shared feelings of the past.

Splitting

On the surface, it may appear as though the couple are very different, perhaps polarised, when in fact, each is carrying unknown aspects of the other's personality. Whilst there is usually conscious condemnation of the other's behaviour, there is also an unconscious identification with it. This explains why an angry man may have married an apparently placid, angelic woman; the two are enmeshed in a 'good one, bad one' kind of relationship, each needing the other to express a hidden side of themselves.

This defensive mechanism of splitting therefore involves unacceptable feelings being denied, projected into the other partner and then disowned. That other partner, in turn, carries and expresses a double dose of that feeling. The couple support the split by collusively preserving the system and mutually perpetuating it.

When this kind of splitting creates an unbearable imbalance in the relationship, as with Klaus and Louise, marital therapy aims to help both partners to understand and acknowledge the denied aspects of themselves which they are projecting into the other.

Between the partners, intrapsychic conflicts are acted out externally in this interpersonal way. When Klaus expressed his depressed feelings, Louise condemned them, avoiding conscious knowledge of her inner identification with such feelings. She could have continued to deny the existence of the same, sad child inside her, but she managed to face and understand some of her own past pain.

Such insight may have precipitated much sadness and depression. However, owning her feelings, sharing the problem and taking back some of the projections from Klaus as the sad, bad one, was the beginning of growth and balance personally and in the relationship.

Photographs can be used in marital therapy to help resolve the split; they may reveal in a gentle way, and more powerfully than words, the fundamental similarities in personality that may be consciously denied. The photograph provided a less threatening way of helping Louise see herself in her husband.

Photographs may be used to illustrate vividly this unconscious mutuality of feeling and agreement behind the tension of opposites in marriage, thus helping to bring a couple closer. Chris and Anita, who were very polarised emotionally, had been struggling in therapy to find some kind of meeting point after years of conflict. They were asked by their therapist to choose three photographs and bring them to therapy, initially without letting each other know of their choice.

Both were amazed – and heartened – to find that they had selected very similar photographs. They had each brought a picture of themselves cradling their first child; this synchronicity was significant to both, in terms of their shared creativity. It also led to a mutual disclosure about their own needs for parenting.

Further images from marital therapy

Melanie and Kevin spoke of sexual problems, where Kevin felt tense and had difficulty in relaxing. Both had experienced a childhood where sex was a taboo subject and parental injunctions against pleasure and individual freedom were strong. Whilst many couples may, figuratively speaking, have their parents sitting at the end of the bed, Kevin actually had family pictures of his parents, looking rather disapprovingly down on the marital bed from the dressing table.

Once they were aware of the roots of their problems, these photographs came to signify to both partners the rigid manner in which they had preserved parental internalisations from childhood, and which were affecting their adult relationship.

A wedding photograph was central in helping Shelley and Graham to understand some of their relationship difficulties. This had pride of place in Graham's parental home and was gradually enlarged over the years. It showed the groom on his wedding day, with his brother, father and mother, but the bride was not pictured. This was the only photograph of the wedding that was in his parents' house.

Shelley saw the photograph as signifying her feelings of not belonging at all in her husband's family, but neither partner had ever dared mention the picture whilst in Graham's parental household. As therapy progressed, both began to realise that it also symbolised the ambivalence in their relationship about growing up and being committed to one another. Neither was sure whether they were child or spouse, having great difficulties with issues of separation and individuation.

Freeze-frame images

Many times in therapy, the interaction between the partners in the here and now is very powerfully expressed in their expressions, postures and body language. The inextricable link between mind and body means that physical, visual images can tell the therapist much about emotional states. With this holistic attitude, she will be able to isolate specific moments in the therapy when a typical interaction is expressed so vividly, so powerfully and in such a dramatic image, that they perfectly express the whole essence of the couple's problem.

The partners form themselves, unconsciously, into a kind of living sculpture of their marital problem. Such moments can be put to excellent therapeutic use, if only they can be captured. If the couple have agreed earlier in the therapy to 'freeze' such a moment for the therapist's polaroid camera, then, perhaps, something of that moment may be preserved on film. Otherwise, the therapist needs to use all her powers of description to convey the nature of the image that she has perceived, to describe the imaginary photograph she has taken.

This crucial, fleeting moment, may, holographically, be a complete reflection of the whole picture of the marital interaction. In identifying such a moment, the therapist may be able to help the couple gain insight into the area in which change is needed. She can subsequently encourage her patients to imagine how the photograph – and their interaction – could have been different.

For example, Karen and Julian's way of relating to each other was summed up in a repetitive freeze-frame image that constantly flashed itself before me in therapy. These were moments of striking visual impact, describing the whole of their initial interaction: Julian would be pleading, accusing and aggressive, leaning towards his wife, pressurising her to speak. Karen would be closed up, hair covering her face, looking down, in a kind of victim stance, arms hugging herself, legs tightly together.

I described the picture before me; when the couple were able to 'see' the image from my description, they began to talk about the feelings beneath the poses. Once the picture has been described, the image can be 'played' with, to enable the couple to gain new ways of seeing. Both recognised for the first time that Julian's way of being was inherited from his father and that Karen used to close up when her mother pressurised her as a child. This use of a real or imaginary photograph helps such comparisons to be made, allowing past and present to be compared. If a real photograph has been taken, this can be kept by the couple, and compared with further interactions as the relationship becomes clearer.

I also suggested to Karen and Julian that we consider reversing the picture in our minds. This was a way of helping them loosen their fixed projections onto each other. The 'photograph' needed to be reframed, turned round, so that we could see the 'negative' side of each partner.

After considerable resistance, Julian began to stop attacking his wife verbally and to reflect introspectively on the part of *himself* that felt like a victim. As he reversed the picture of himself, Karen began to look up at him, to be more active and verbal, changing her physical stance. She slowly risked verbalising some feelings. There began to be an external reversal, and this must have been reflective of the internal.

In time, as they both began to take more responsibility for themselves and to change repetitive patterns of relating to each other, they were able to act more autonomously, become separate, and more loving. And, almost imperceptibly, the 'photograph' before me changed dramatically. Now I could 'capture' them, repeatedly, relating easily and equally;

physically their interacting selves formed a much more balanced shape, with both leaning back comfortably in their chairs, legs crossed towards each other. This made a very pleasing pattern aesthetically, balanced and synchronous, reflecting the new atmosphere of harmony and symmetry in their relationship.

This more active way of working with couples encourages a flexible attitude, enabling fluidity in a couple's relatedness, so that rigid forms of interaction may begin to move and change.

FAMILY DYNAMICS AND INTERACTION AND HOW THESE ARE MANIFESTED IN THE PHOTOGRAPH

Let us now move from a visual exploration of marriage into the wider context of family interaction and the photograph, venturing further into the complex world of family images. Here we shall begin to discover how such pictures may help the therapist to understand and recognise the recurring themes, the universal issues that confound many families, the pathological systems that create interminable mayhem and deadlock for the individuals trapped within them.

Whilst I work with a broadly psychoanalytic approach, I have found that a knowledge of the theory of family systems is also helpful when looking for family dynamics within the photograph. The two approaches are often combined by marital and family therapists, and this combination may be effective when looking at family photographs.

Systems theory regards any interaction or behaviour within the family as created and maintained by every member of that family. Each individual is a component part of that whole system, which is founded upon a complex interplay of entwined relationships, with its own rules and structure. Thus, change in one part of the family system influences the whole of that system.

In utilising some of the main concepts of systems theory, the therapist will be able to help her patients journey beyond the superficial images and to enter into the deeper realms of family interaction.

In any quest for insight, it is essential that problems, themes and issues are *seen* – and acknowledged – by the patient. Photographs help dramatically in this seeing, bringing family interactions sharply into focus, sometimes confirming, sometimes contradicting, memory and perception. Aspects of the family's functioning and organisation may be unconsciously acted out on camera, providing for future generations a lasting record of its pathology.

In order to be able to readily identify family themes and issues, it is important to have some understanding of some of the patterns and dynamics that typically occur within the family group. These are plentiful, and must be examined in detail.

The family myth

The therapist needs to have an understanding of the existence of family myths, and an awareness of how they are reflected in many family albums. Otherwise, there is a danger that she may be misled by their powerful falsifications.

The family album can reflect the family's myths. From its silent pages there emerges a voice that utters with certainty: 'This is our family.' Whatever may subsequently happen to that family, whatever rifts, vendettas, feuds, splits and losses may occur to rend it apart, the family album doggedly signifies and affirms that it once *was*, it existed as an entity.

Here bonds are maintained that may long since have been dissolved; these photographs therefore sustain a stereotyped, fixed image of the family that, although partial and incomplete, is powerfully compelling and pervasive.

Milgram (1977: 350) has said: '. . . a photograph does not only record events. It creates them.' With the camera, the family manufactures the kind of images that it desires, lifting selected scenarios from life and presenting them as a whole story, inevitably creating in this way an intricate and seductive fantasy.

There is apparently little to contradict the likely story of the family album; through its myths, perpetuated by a host of persistently selective images, we are persuasively urged to believe its lively half-truths. But if we dare to look overleaf, as it were, to the other side of the snap-happiness, to the world of the negative, we will see the dark reflections of a shadow-land. These are images that often steal into the family album by 'mistake', the unnoticed gestures or expressions that only a skilled photographic reader would perceive.

Photographs that conceal: the importance of the narrative

In view of the fact that the camera can obscure, limit and distort reality, and because the family tends to make use of this fact, it is necessary to pause and reconsider the importance of a reliable accompanying narrative whilst exploring family pictures. However careful and persistent may be one's scrutiny of the family album, the corroboration and confirmation of an informed verbal account is essential if real truths are to be discovered. For, when the camera belies these truths, the verbal explanation will penetrate beyond the smiles.

Often, this explanation is so opposite to what is revealed in the photograph, that we may be highly disturbed by the ability of the camera to conceal. We will become painfully aware of the power of the family to create its visual myths.

Laura produced a photograph of her family that graphically illustrated this point. It showed her as a child of 5, with her mother and two sisters. All of them were smiling 'happily'. The children wore little white peaked bonnets.

Mother appeared to be proudly displaying her daughters for the camera, holding their hands. The older child, on the left of mother, held her youngest sister's shoulders from behind, also smiling. Mother wore a smart coat, with a hood, and her dark, wavy hair shone from beneath it. She looked an attractive and benign figure, with soft, full cheeks and clear skin. They were standing in a garden, with a blossom tree behind them. A perfect family picture. . . . Now let us hear what Laura had to say in connection with her photograph:

> At around the time of this photograph, I was extremely unhappy because Mother was already putting me in rooms on bread and water. I remember that there was an inquisition about an ink stain on a cloth – I denied I had done it – she took me up to her room and beat me. She said that she couldn't punish me enough in one go, so she'd come back in a certain number of hours. She beat me with a riding whip, or a wooden spoon, or a breadboard. Later on she boasted quite proudly that she had cured me of telling lies by this method.

Laura's upbringing was catalogue of pain and physical abuse, in the guise of 'parenting'. But the photograph reflects only the family's public face, upholding the happiness myth. Jo Spence has said: 'The family album tells the story from the adults' point of view. They seem to be saying – "Look, we did the best we could for you."'[1]

In such photographs, therefore, it is only an informed narrative that can then reveal the disturbing dissonance between what is seen and what is really happening.

'A living cliché . . .'

The family often creates its myths, or defensive distortions of reality, in order to avoid having to face unpleasant facts or feelings. Using a photographic image, the family therapist Ferreira has described the family myth itself as:

> . . . a living cliché, an animated album of family pictures that no one quite dares to erase or throw away, essential as they are to the legitimization and consecration of the ongoing relationship.
>
> (Ferreira 1963: 460)

The photograph album helps to develop and preserve such myths, highlighting the family's fervent attempts to present itself in the best possible light. The family thus uses its photograph album to support and maintain such fabrications, to present itself in bright colours and fixed images. These hide the truth, and often may keep the family fixed in an unhealthy set:

> Family mythology consists of all those shared family images and stories which help give the family its continuing identity, but which under close inspection, are judged to be highly coloured. They are, as it were, seen through tinted spectacles, like the man who was perceived as extra strong, despite his heart failing, or the decorated 'war hero' grandfather, who never in fact saw any action.
>
> To return to the analogy of colour. Any one particular colour is created by filtering out the remainder of the light spectrum. If this filtering is too extensive, mythology no longer acts as colourful heraldry, but as a restrictive set of blinkers. As Ferreira (1963) points out all families need some mythology, but too much deadens.
>
> Myths about the present consist of attributions of certain roles to certain members of the family, e.g. 'crazy one', with all the accompanying expectations. These images become established because they are not challenged. Sometimes the whole family may be seen in monochrome; e.g. rose-tinted for a 'happy family'. In other families each character is seen in sharp contrast, e.g. 'black sheep' and pure white 'saints'.
>
> To support these consensus images, stories are told to illustrate how their forebears, and they themselves behaved in a way which led to the present state of affairs. This past and present mythology is interdependent. The family's current view of itself may change. In that case the past will also have to be seen in a new light. The family stories will be given a new twist. This process is called editing and re-editing the past.
>
> (Byng-Hall 1979: 103–4)

The family album may also be used in therapy, however, to dispel these mythical contrivances that have been manufactured over the years. It provides graphic evidence of their existence, thus rendering them available for scrutiny and reassessment. Through using photographs therapeutically, the family can learn to identify hitherto uncompromising fictions, to trace them through the generations, and subsequently to 're-edit' them in the light of truth.

Myths are perpetuated through a lack of awareness and understanding; the photograph, used therapeutically, can help the patient towards new insight, offering up the questionable images for examination. Thus therapist and patient will learn to query the happy one-sidedness of the album and, as we shall subsequently see, to recognise the many subtle signs within it that indicate the presence of these defensive family myths. A well-thumbed family album may thus take on a whole new set of meanings, which may reveal in a hopeful way how we have grown and developed. But such a second look can also be painful and disturbing.

Juliet was still grieving for a marriage that she had thought idyllic. Her husband had left her the previous year after having an affair with her best friend. Juliet began to see new aspects in old photographs from the family album. She now noticed that her husband was always standing by the side of his lover, who, as Juliet's friend, was pictured frequently with their family. Juliet had looked at those pictures many times during the marriage, and had never noticed the couple's closeness before: 'And I never saw it at the time, either. That reflects how I did not know what was happening in the marriage.'

As Juliet looked back at her pictures, she spotted disturbing truths that had been there all the time, beneath the smiles and the 'happy' family scenes. This helped her realise that she had created a myth for herself, and that, in many ways, she was grieving the loss of a fantasy.

Whilst such photographs as I have described above may function to conceal the truth, in many cases, photographs can be considerably more overt in their revelations, imparting much that is significant. Using the family album, it is possible to trace relationship patterns through the generations, in order that the patient may be helped to alter the destructive patterns and to recognise, value and maintain the healthy ones.

A look at family roles and structures

It often appears on photographs that some people seem to have protective functions, whilst others are clearly being protected. Photographs may reveal evidence of the kinds of roles adopted by individual members within the structure of the family system. Some children, for instance, have to play onerous adult roles from an early age.

Betty, who saw herself as having been a parental child, showed me a photograph which very much illustrated her function within the family and, indeed, within her parents' marriage. Betty was the eldest child of three, the only girl. Unconsciously, and collusively, she acted out from an early age the repeated family myth that the first-born female must take the parental child role. It was she who felt responsible for her parents' welfare, especially in terms of their marriage, in which she was supporter to her mother, often staying off school to comfort, help and advise her. She also attempted to be the peacemaker in her parents' frenzied arguments.

In this particular photograph, where the family were posing for a seaside photographer, Betty, aged 13, stood in the centre. This physical centrality represented her pivotal position at the nucleus of the family – for she was the child who seemed to hold it together. She had her arms around the waist of each parent, with father on her right, mother on her left. She appeared to be almost physically supporting both of them, smiling a stoic smile, but with heavy, tired eyes, that looked too knowing, too responsible for a child of 13. It was Betty to whom mother came with her problems about her violent husband. It was Betty whom father used as a go-between when he and his wife were not on speaking terms.

In the photograph, the youngest child stood beside his mother, who clutched him possessively, the anxious firmness in her grip betraying her own unmet needs for nurture. Betty felt that her younger brother would have been relieved to be at the opposite end of the picture from father, who angrily envied him all the maternal attention. The middle brother stood on the other side, at his father's right hand, his firmly favoured child.

The photograph demonstrates a confusion and a precariousness in the family structure. There is no evidence of a clear boundary between adults and children, only a feeling of muddled roles, indeterminate limits, a lack of differentiation. The photograph exactly reflects the situation in this enmeshed family, where there was little separation between the parents and the children.

In contrast to the above, consider Dr Patricia Love's description of the boundary in a healthy family:

> This boundary can be likened to a one-way valve. It allows the adults to meet the needs of the children, but it prevents the children from meeting the needs of the adults. Although love and affection flow freely in both directions, the children are not allowed to become part of the adult support system.
>
> (Love 1990: 97)

Meaningful differences

The photograph can also can further reveal aspects of family dynamics, through highlighting the polarisations, contradictions, differences and paradoxes within the family. Through them, we can see for ourselves how one 'different' individual, standing out starkly from the rest, may have taken on and expressed various behaviours and feelings for the others in the family.

There are many ways to appear the 'odd one out' in a photograph. One way is through dress. Mark looks strikingly at odds with the rest of his family in the album; he wears exaggerated punk clothes whilst his family is most conventional in its dress and attitudes.

Photograph 18 shows the considerable contrast between Mark and his parents in physical terms. This reflects the contrast in terms of outlook. Mark comments:

> I don't mind what people think about me. Mum always keeps a smile on her face, though. She is trying to keep up appearances; they matter to her. They don't matter at all to me. I want to introduce some fun into the conventionality around me. I want a pacifist rebellion.

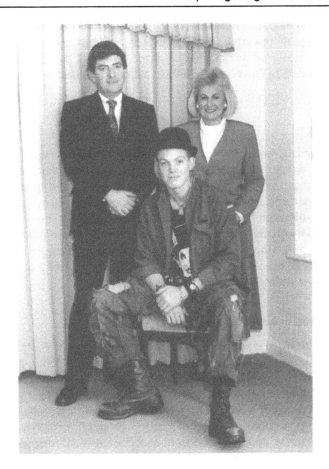

Photograph 18

Mark's mother, however, is able to admit to some envy of her son's dramatic ability to flout convention, feeling that she certainly could not make such an overt statement. Perhaps he is, therefore, expressing the need to be different on behalf of the whole family, symbolising it in physical terms.

As we leaf through the family album, it is therefore important to remember that noticeable dissimilarities on a physical level may reveal much about the emotional load that an individual may be carrying for other family members. We saw in Chapter 2 how Diana's expression differed so much from that of her family; she alone was unsmiling. This gave clues to a deep and ongoing family problem, where Diana seemed to carry the 'negative' projections for the others and was regarded as wayward and rebellious.

The words of Carl Jung are relevant here:

Generally speaking, all the life which the parents could have lived, but of which they thwarted themselves for artificial motives, is passed on to the children in substitute form. Hence it is that excessively moral-minded parents have what are called 'unmoral' children. . . .

(Jung 1977: 191)

Scapegoating

Sometimes one person, often a child, is scapegoated in this way, frequently labelled mad or bad. In other photographs, the 'scapegoat' or 'black sheep' will be set apart, partially hidden by others, or even missing altogether.

At the other end of the spectrum, it is possible to recognise a highly favoured family member, perhaps a child, who carries the 'good' label. This can be an equally burdensome position, for the chosen child may feel the pressure of having to live up to impossible parental expectations. This child appears to be always the centre of attention in family photographs, whereas other siblings seem somehow out of focus.

Triangular relationships

Evidence of triangular situations is often abundant in family albums, which frequently show how one person is being excluded from an inimate twosome. Often this person is the scapegoat. On some photographs, mother and child, or children, are closely allied, and father is peripheral. Or it may be mother who is set apart, hardly able to get a look-in.

For a vivid example of some of the above-mentioned dynamics, and to enable a more detailed exploration of repetitively unhealthy family patterns through photographs, let us now return to Klaus, whose family album contained a series of most significant pictures. Through these, he was able to identify some of the models of relating within marriage and family that had persisted through generations. He saw how they stretched far back into his past, manifesting themselves in the lives of his ancestors before his birth and reaching right through to the lives of his children. He began to understand the roots of the problems he had had, especially his tendency to be critically cold and his fear of intimacy.

Take a long look at Photograph 19, to discover the evidence within it of a real family problem. Here we see Klaus's maternal grandmother, together with his mother, aunt and uncle as children. What can you notice about the positioning, the stances, the expressions? What information can you glean from these about possible relationships and attitudes?

Klaus had other photographs of the same group of people, taken on different days and different occasions, which, strikingly, reveal the same triangular patterns. Notice the way in which the three females are standing on the right side of the picture, separated from the boy by a larger space.

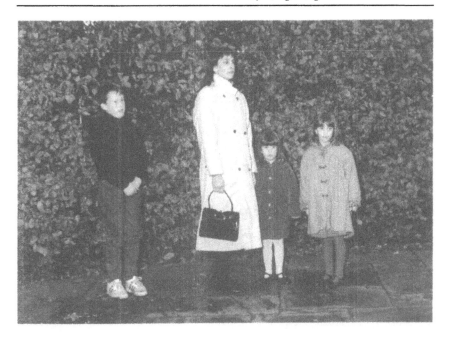

Photograph 19
Posed by models

The boy appears to be very much set apart from his family. His body-language is stiffer than that of his sisters; he seems less relaxed than they.

See how the two sisters are close to each other physically, almost touching, forming together one point of the triangle, and how the mother is turned away from her son, towards them. Mother appears oblivious of him, focusing on the exclusive relationship with her girls. She almost shields them with her body; certainly they cannot be seen by their brother, and he is seen by no one in the picture. Klaus's narrative exactly confirmed what the photograph suggests, for his uncle was excluded by his family, who labelled him as the black sheep, whilst the two girls were the pride and joy of their parents.

The visual triangulation in this photograph revealed much about the family system; it also symbolised for Klaus the ongoing coldness within the family, the conditional love and the emphasis on the need to achieve high standards. Klaus had inherited the family difficulty with closeness and it expressed itself in his marital relationship.

Repeated patterns

Most significantly, photographs of his mother and stepfather, Frank, helped Klaus to identify the patterns he had repeated in his present

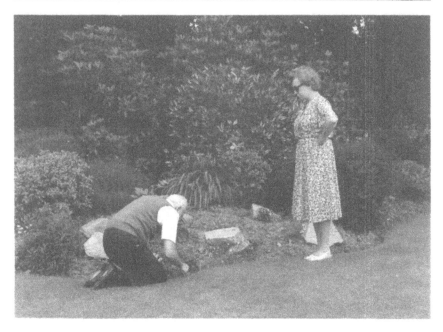

Photograph 20
Posed by models

relationships. In Photograph 20, Mother is standing over Frank, as he plants some flowers. Klaus related:

> The issue of class had been a pervading theme in my mother's family for generations. You can see it in many of these pictures. Mother was unhappy and fault-finding, because she felt that Frank was not up to her class. This photograph in the garden sums up their relationship. He's on his knees before her. She was criticising him there. I remember – I took the photo. She'd also stand above us in the kitchen whilst we were eating and she'd start criticising. My grandmother did this as well – she had a power thing, she always stood at breakfast, admonishing my grandfather; she never gave him a moment's peace. This picture could represent either generation, both followed the same patterns. Come to think of it, I really hate it if my wife stands whilst I'm eating. I get the same feelings of being criticised. It feels so cold and uncaring.

In Photograph 21 Klaus's mother is again with his stepfather in the garden. Klaus explained:

> My stepfather always wanted to please my mother, but never could. In this picture, you can see a frequent pose of hers, and a very familiar look. Sort of gazing away, superior, cut-off. I recognise that I do that

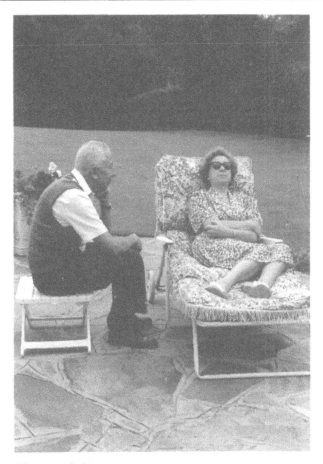

Photograph 21
Posed by models

now, to people in my family. He is looking at her and thinking – 'My God, I try.' I know that look of his. I've repeated this picture time and time again with my wife.

For Klaus, the pattern of one partner visibly cutting off or showing discomfort with closeness, or separate from an enthusiastic other, had traced itself right through his life and is strikingly mirrored in his photograph album. For example, Klaus would repeatedly be pictured looking at mother, but she would stare wistfully into space, posing as she had been taught as a child, seemingly unaware of his needy gaze.

To see just how much this pattern has been repeated from one generation to another, compare Photographs 21 and 22. The latter now shows Klaus and his wife. Notice how Klaus's glum, critical expression

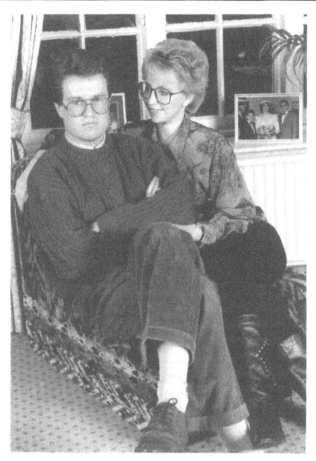

Photograph 22
Posed by models

mirrors that of his mother, and how his wife, Louise, looks at him, almost imploringly, just as Frank had looked at his spouse. Klaus recollected how Louise could never be right, and how he excluded her, just as his mother did his stepfather.

As Klaus looked again at the pictures of his mother and stepfather in their garden, he was reminded of the way he had related to his own children.

> I used to make intimidating threats to my family, just as mother did to me. The garden pictures bring that back. I remember an episode where I intimidated my willing child when gardening. Now she won't do anything for me. It is very sad and painful; but I understand it now.

Klaus had projected his own internal, abused child into his daughter, and then emotionally abused that child within her. As he looked at those pictures, he had a sense of lost opportunity and was sad that his daughter seemed to be repeating some of the patterns of intimidation and criticism with her boyfriend. He felt some despair at not being able to go back and make reparation to her, although he had attempted to do this in the present.

Klaus suddenly noticed that, in the series of photographs of his elder daughter, she did not look happy. She was hardly ever smiling. He saw that this reflected how he too appeared on photographs as a child, and that the pattern stretched back through his mother to his grandmother and, most likely, beyond. He reflected:

> We gave our daughter a lot materially, *but we did not make her smile.* I can see this through the pictures, though I know it in myself. It's brought it home to me, seeing her not smiling in those photographs. I feel very guilty. But, at least she has a parent who's seen it, I didn't have. What can I do now? . . . It's perhaps a pointer to the future . . .

Perhaps most importantly in terms of his understanding of his marital relationship, Klaus was able to remember and perceive through his photographs that, whilst his mother had been happy when she and Frank were courting, within a few months, mother was saying she had made a dreadful mistake. In retrospect, it was even apparent on the photograph taken at his mother's wedding to Frank that there were the signs of potential future discord. The photograph shows the bride and groom sitting together. Klaus's mother is arm in arm with her new husband, but she is leaning right away from him, tilting her head as far away as possible. Head tilting *towards* a person may signify affection, but in this picture, Klaus's mother is very definitely giving a message of distance.

Whilst at the time, this head tilting on the wedding photograph may have gone unnoticed, hindsight showed that it had some significance and meaning in the light of subsequent events in terms of the couple's relationship.

It dawned on Klaus, looking at the photographs, and seeing the contrasts in mood and attitude before and after his mother's marriage, that the pattern was exactly the same for him. There were happy, romantic pictures of the early relationship with Louise, but this happiness soon disappeared, to be replaced by the old pattern of one partner sitting at the feet of the other, who is critical and unaffectionate. This repeated pattern, which he traced through his family album, helped Klaus understand some of the family messages that he had unconsciously received about marriage and enabled a change in the inner picture of marriage that he had inherited.

The use of photographs in family therapy

As in individual and marital therapy, photographs enable families in therapy to recognise patterns of interaction and to gain insight into the family system and their role in it.

They also help people to get 'in touch' with members of their extended family, and those who have died or disappeared from the family scene. Photographs may be used to revivify feelings and memories, so that these can be shared and discussed. They reveal changes in the family and the individuals within it over the years. There is also provided a stimulus to interact, to discuss the images, share memories, both within the session, and outside therapy. As family members begin to approach others outside for photographs, there is often a restoration of relationships that may have lapsed or deteriorated.

In family therapy, past experiences are revisited through snapshots of earlier experiences. Only in the setting of the family can children and parents remember the past together, so that each can better hear the other. Then, the feelings and thoughts about the experience depicted in the photograph may be shared and discussed within the safe boundary of the therapy.

Family therapists may use photographs in innovative and interesting ways, to help their patients learn more about their family problems and develop strategies for change.

Corbit (in Wadeson *et al.* 1989: 285) helps her families to recreate their problems through photographs, by first having each member pose for the camera in any way they choose. Then the images are cut out and the family pastes them on a board, using art materials to create a background. Whilst they are engaged in this, the therapist watches their interaction very carefully, for this is full of symbolic clues. The members are also encouraged to construct photographs of how they would like their family to be, posing the other members to fit their ideal picture.

Zilbach (1986) has used simulated photographs of families in therapy to enhance her writing on the subject. These gave a sense of immediacy in her descriptions of the therapeutic process, and were useful in conveying aspects of the interaction not easily described in words. These photographs were then also used in supervision and case conferences.

Entin comments on the significance of 'favourite photographs' and how they can be revealing in family therapy:

> Favorite pictures of one's self, spouse, children and parents are significant in helping to understand each person's view of the emotional process operating at the time within self and family. Favorite pictures are interesting because they have both visual and non-visual referents. Visually they refer to a characteristic look or expression, while their non-visual referents are about remembrances of times, events, people, places. Obviously, there will not be unanimous agreement about which pictures best represent the family, although in highly fused families they may all tend to 'think alike' and attempt to agree on their selections.
>
> (Entin 1982: 210)

This chapter has focused on the family album as an aid to the therapeutic process, examining also aspects of the theory and practice of marital and family therapy.

In the next chapter, we move out of the context of marriage and the family into the wider world, to see who else may benefit from the therapeutic use of photographs.

Chapter 7

Who can benefit?

Photographs furnish instant history, instant sociology, instant participation.
(Sontag 1987: 75)

We have seen in the previous chapters how photographs can be used with patients in therapy as a tool to help promote growth and change; let us now widen our exploration of the use of the medium and venture further afield to meet some of the different groups of people who can benefit from photographs in various therapeutic settings.

REMINISCENCE THERAPY

Reminiscence therapy may be used in many group situations where there is a need to stimulate interest and communication. Within psychiatric day hospitals, for example, photographs and other memorabilia help to enhance self-image, encourage group interaction and help people to tell their stories.

In work with the elderly, reminiscence therapy aims to reduce the deterioration of intellectual and social skills, through stimulating memory and enabling conversation. Books, clothes, old coins, war memorabilia and other objects are used to promote recall and discussion in a group setting. In addition, music, taste and smells may further assist reminiscence. Photographs play a most vital part in this kind of therapy, enabling a conversation to begin and putting memories into a visual context.

As people grow older, they begin to reminisce naturally; many younger people may find this kind of recollective musing difficult to hear and tend to dismiss it as an indication of decline. But such repetitive retelling can represent a valuable and therapeutic attempt to connect with the past, to resolve old conflicts and perhaps to come to terms with thoughts of death: 'In some individuals, the frequently repeated tales of the past are similar to the repetition, remembering and working-through sequences observed in the psychoanalytic treatment situation' (Pollock 1981: 280).

Reminscence therapy can be an enjoyable way of reaching others; it also helps to confirm identity, and provides evidence and reassurance that the past existed, at a time when the present may feel vague and confused.

With their unique ability to stimulate memory, photographs also play an especially invaluable part in therapy with those who have memory problems, such as victims of Alzheimer's Disease, senile dementia and other forms of amnesia.

Working with dementia: Fox Ward

My visit to Fox Ward, Sutton Hospital, Surrey, one bright winter afternoon, showed me how important is the use of photographs for those with memory and communication problems. Here, dedicated staff attended to patients suffering from dementia.

Some patients dozed in armchairs; others trod aimless paths through the corridor, backwards, forwards, endlessly, compulsively. Some stared blankly, others talked in words that were confused and confusing. Yet there was a pervading sense of comfortable community in this bright ward, and a hopefulness that emanated from the staff and many of the patients.

The walls were lined with photographs; at the entrance to the ward were colourful images of the staff, to assist patients and visitors. Display boards beside each patient's bed were pinned with photographs of themselves and their families; these helped strengthen a sense of identity and gave value and importance. Mirrors were also strategically placed around the ward, so that patients could catch confirming reflections of themselves.

There were pictures of past public events and many of the royal family. Photographs of Christmas and birthday parties in the ward had been taken with polaroid cameras, as the immediate results benefited those with poor short-term memory.

Such patients cannot be taught new material; the aim of reminiscence therapy is to reinforce long-term memory. This will enhance self-esteem and confidence, in that relating personal stories about the past will not expose short-term memory loss. In this way, patients are spared embarrassment and a feeling of being deskilled and threatened. Disruptive or unusual behaviour is also reduced because the patient is absorbed and occupied, whilst feeling heard and accepted.

Each patient in Fox Ward had a life album, a book of family photographs which had been made with the help of relatives. One such album belonged to Daisy, a diminutive and very old lady who sat hunched, curled up, tiny in a large armchair. Daisy was unable to speak and appeared to be unavailable emotionally to anyone who tried to reach her.

Unavailable, that is, until a nurse, familiar to Daisy, showed her the photograph album. Because she did not respond to words, questions and comments had to be written down for her. As the pages were turned, Daisy lifted her head slightly and gave a fragile smile of recognition. She then began to make loud sounds that were recognisable as words and names only to those who knew her well. She seemed to come alive when she saw the pictures, stimulated into awareness, revealing her very evident sense of humour.

Through the photographs, the staff in Fox Ward were helped to learn more about the patients and their lives, past and present. They were able to reach people who otherwise showed few signs of communicating; thus the albums proved to be mutually beneficial, encouraging trust and understanding. It was essential for the staff to know the patients really well, because sometimes a flicker of recognition was the only response. But, no matter how indistinct this response was, the telling of such stories was a most important factor in preserving identity and self-esteem. The albums were a living history book, a kind of 'This is your life' in pictures, some of them going back a hundred and fifty years. When the patient died, the album was given to the family as a lasting memory and tribute.

Amnesia

For patients who suffer from amnesia resulting from brain injury through illness or accident, photographs can help to restore a vanished sense of self. Where there is no memory of the past, the images can help to show patients their own life and to build up a picture of themselves. This functions to enhance self-esteem and gives some feeling of identity.

THE USE OF PHOTOGRAPHS WITH CHILDREN AND ADOLESCENTS

Photographs have been utilised with considerable success at the other end of the age spectrum. In therapy with children, photographs may be taken and used therapeutically to help children tell their story. Sand pictures, meaningfully created during play therapy, may be photographed to preserve them for future reference and confirmation. Difficult scenarios are reconstructed in the sand, using toys and figures to express aspects of the internal world.

Irene Corbit has combined photography and sandtray work with a 6-year-old child, suffering from profound fears:

> In a recent session, Holly began a sandtray. Corbit asked her if she would like to put herself in the sandtray. 'How can I do that?' Holly asked. 'We'll take a "brave" picture of you, and put the picture into the tray,' Corbit answered. Holly posed for the instant picture in which she was to feel brave. The photograph was cut out, mounted, and a stand was then glued onto the back of the figure. The sandtray contained many frightening figures, but 'brave' Holly stood up to them.

We then took an instant photograph of the sandtray so that Holly could have her own copy of the scene.

(in Wadeson *et al.* 1989: 282)

Subsequently, Holly's fears did reduce, for she had felt more in control through such work with her therapist.

For a child whose life may have been uncertain and disrupted, a therapist's holiday breaks may be an unbearable reminder of past feelings of abandonment. A photograph of the therapist or playroom can function as a transitional object for the child during the therapist's absence. In a similar way, at the end of therapy, patient and therapist can exchange photographs as part of the leaving process.[1] Some therapists may, however, view this as a controversial and questionable practice, regarding the giving of photographs to a patient as a collusive way of denying feelings about the therapist's absence, or about the end of therapy.

Therapists who teach children of all ages to print their own photographs have commented on the therapeutic value of this task. Developing the photographs, and being an instigator of the magical process of photography, gives confidence. The process here may be seen as an end in itself – catharsis through creativity. Such photographic acts of self-expression may quite often represent a first-time experience for children, as they photograph and are photographed by others. All this gives them a sense of self-esteem, responsibility and importance as individuals. Having themselves photographed also means that they become centre-stage, attracting much-needed attention and focus.

Often, photo-therapy with troubled adolescents is active rather than passive, in order to engage patients who may otherwise lose interest and concentration. In many cases, the making and taking of the pictures provides a symbolic way of manipulating and ruling the world, giving a feeling of empowerment and self-worth. As photographs are taken and people asked to pose, considerable learning takes place about self and other, in an accepting atmosphere.

There is an excitement in such work, a gaining of new skills and a sense of creative fun as the pictures are developed and magically take shape. This is a safe and non-threatening way to engage resistant adolescents, who may prove unresponsive to other therapeutic techniques. The 'once-removed' quality of the photograph facilitates a reassuring distance for the adolescent afraid of intimacy.

The kind of conversation that photographs permit proved especially helpful in the experience of one teacher of emotionally disturbed adolescents. She shared her own personal photographs with her students, and this encouraged them to do the same:

One 13-year-old-boy who was living in a residential facility had made no friends in the class until he started using the pictures to show what he was unable to tell about his parents and his real home. Ms Turner [the teacher] explains: 'Children with limited communication skills had found another means of contacting others and opening up to them.'

(McKinney 1979: 29)

The use of photographs to enhance self-image

Research in America has shown that photographs can help in the enhancement of the self-esteem in children and adolescents. Ammerman and Fryrear conducted a study which centred on body image:

> . . . with the assumption that an enhancement in body image produces a corresponding enhancement in self-esteem behaviour. It was further assumed that children with low self-esteem have a distorted body image and that accurate feedback of the children's appearances would result in an enhancement of body image. Photography was chosen as the feedback method.

(Ammerman and Fryrear 1975: 320)

This method was found to be a valuable one, enabling discussion about feelings and self-image. Further research, with a similar aim, centred around photographing adolescent social interactions, such as shaking hands, offering cigarettes, playing cards (Fryrear *et al.* 1977).

Hogan uses exercises with photographs to improve self-image in 'client groups with various learning disabilities, emotional disorders and physical handicaps'. She outlines the goals of her work with photographs: '1) to have children understand their feelings and perception of themselves, and 2) to have the children develop a beginning awareness of the possible relationship between self-image and behavior' (Hogan 1981: 195).

The exercises involve the children in photographing each other and then exploring feelings about the resulting images of self, other and environment. Photographs are also taken of 'important things' – articles that are 'prized' or 'treasured' – and the children are encouraged to make a 'picture book of me'. Specific themes are introduced, to be expressed through photographs, such as 'when I grow up and other fantasies'. In addition, a range of feelings is identified and acted out for the camera, and this is followed by a discussion of the finished results.

Children in care and those who are to be adopted

Photographs and life-story books help to establish some continuity for children in care, whose experiences will have inevitably induced some psychological fragmentation. Social workers are aware of the importance of building a picture of the past with such children, who also gain a sense of control and a feeling of co-operative creativity with their worker through making life-albums. These will contain written, drawn and photographic information about the child's life.

Additionally, photographs play a most important part in many of the stages involved in the adoption process. Sometimes, photographs of children are initially put in a newspaper, to help find adoptive parents.

Once an adoption has been planned, family photographs may be given to the child, perhaps a couple of days before the child meets the new parents. These will provide something for the child to have and to look at at this early and delicate stage in the process. The giving of such pictures does need to be done sensitively, with an awareness of timing and of the impact on the child.

Some prospective parents are asked to make a photograph album of their home and family, to familiarise the child prior to such an important and possibly overwhelming meeting, and also to act as a bridging object into a new life. One such album was intriguingly crafted out of felt, the whole fitting into a zip bag. Inside, were clever little pockets and press-studs, which, when opened, revealed friendly introductory messages and pictures of the house, car, family members and its animals. The child carried this bag around before he met the adoptive family; it became very meaningful and precious.

Foster parents can also use this sort of album to help children move on to the adoptive home. In another way, it may also be used by foster parents to delineate the family to which the child really belongs, thus helping to diminish some inevitable confusion.

Adoptive families may use photographs to bring the history of their family to the child, so that the child is not excluded from shared memories. One family inserted pictures of their adopted child into their family album before he arrived at the new home; thus when the child was shown the album, he was already a part of it.

When a child goes to a new family, there is often a desire on the part of that family for the child to 'forget' the past. But social workers try to encourage the adoptive family to supply information as soon as the child starts talking about the natural family, for such memories do need to be recognised and valued. They give the new parents as much written and photographic information as possible about the child's family and past; young children tend to need cues, like photographs, to help them reminisce.

In a similar way, the natural parents will have photographs of their children, to enable them to hold onto memories. Sometimes, after the adoption, the natural parents will ask for photographs of their children as they grow up; this is possible only if the adoptive parents agree.

LEARNING DIFFICULTIES AND PHYSICAL HANDICAP

For both adults and children who may find verbal communication difficult, photographs can provide a way through, a bridge to connect handicapped people with those around them. For people who are deaf, or recovering from a stroke, for those suffering from schizophrenia or autism or for those with other physical or psychological disablements, the photograph can be used, in many different ways, to close the gap and enable some kind of link to be made.

For adults with learning difficulties, once again the use of life-story books helps them to value their achievements, reinforce their memories and increase self-esteem. They contribute to an awareness of family relationships, and activity around photographs, such as discussion and inserting captions, encourages creative thought.

In the case of adults leaving a psychiatric hospital, life-story books have also been used to acknowledge and value a past after long hospital stays, sometimes of thirty or forty years. Photographs may be taken of the rooms in which former patients have spent their lives, and of objects and people who may have been important. If there are no childhood pictures, the patients are encouraged to choose substitutes from magazines.

Photographs enable people who are physically disabled to explore feelings about themselves and their handicaps, and to look at the kind of labels that are put upon them. Pictures taken by disabled people can help the therapist see their world-view:

> One photograph taken by a wheelchair subject was particularly dramatic. The photograph showed twelve persons at a range of about three feet to fifteen feet in a crowd situation, yet no one in the photograph showed eye contact. In fact, the people in view appear to be straining to avoid eye contact with the handicapped person. And in another similar photograph taken in a crowd, again no person makes eye contact, but a large dog near the photogapher has the temerity to look at a person in a wheelchair.
>
> (Ziller and Smith 1977: 178)

ART THERAPY AND THE PHOTOGRAPH

In his work with children with special needs, art therapist Roger Arguile used his camera therapeutically with Charles, aged 6, who had a severe speech disorder. His aim was to visually represent Charles's statements and conversations through the medium of art and photography. Thus, he has taken photographs of Charles using sign-language to spell his name, and to communicate whole sentences. This process helped to preserve creative moments and to encourage language development and communication:

> I responded to Charles and his language problem from my standpoint as an artist. My concern was representing language in terms of visual art. My subject for this was Charles and the verbal and non-verbal

language he spoke was the raw material I used to create the final
drawings and photographic pieces.

(Arguile 1990: 205–6)

. . . he was finding the words to match his powerful language, and I was
seeking to reveal an art language to match his words. A dual creative
process.

(Arguile 1990: 207–8)

Some art therapists encourage people to combine photographs with their
paintings. Such a blending of the different media enables the 'reality' of
the photograph to be contrasted with the fantasy of the painting, so that
these two can be compared and contrasted as they mix and merge into one
image.

Fryrear and Corbit use art therapy and photography, together with other
therapeutic methods, to create 'a multimodal arts approach':

The *visual transitions* procedure features a blending of visual arts,
photography, movement, video, and verbal psychotherapy or group
process. It focusses on providing group members or individual clients
with experiential exercises that allow them to observe, through photographs of themselves, their present state (indicating some type of
rigidity or constriction) and also a more preferred state (indicating a
new level of coping or openness). The still photography and the artwork
are combined to reveal new relationships between these two facets of
the self.

(Fryrear and Corbit 1989: 275)

Sometimes, patients with some artistic ability have brought to therapy
paintings of relatives that they themselves have done after studying their
photographs. They are using the photographs for information, as a basis
for an interpretive painting. It is then interesting to note the differences
between the paintings and the photographs.

Jack, for example, painted pictures of his parents from photographs; his
paintings made them look much uglier than they really had been. Their
eyes looked quite menacing. Into his work he had incorporated the anger
and destructive feelings that he felt towards them; the paintings also
showed something of the way in which he had seen them as a child.

PSYCHODRAMA AND THE PHOTOGRAPH

There are many ways in which photographs are used in psychodrama.
Group members can be asked to bring in a photograph of childhood; they
can then be encouraged to act out the picture and make a living scene of
it, with the help of other members of the group. If there are no
photographs available, members can be asked to imagine a family

photograph that would capture the essence of the family, and describe it or act it out. This imaginary picture, which may fill a gap in the album, can be preserved through the use of a polaroid camera.

These exercises may provoke much emotion. In addition, where members' personal and family photographs are concerned, real or imaginary, it is common for memories and feelings to be triggered by the photographs of others.

Stories and fantasies can be created around such photographs – both one's own and another's. The group may be asked to imagine that they are walking into the photograph and that the people in it are coming to life. They may choose to change the picture, to reconstruct it, either in fantasy, or in reality, recreating the photograph with a real camera.

Some psychodramatists bring into the session their own cut-out newspaper pictures and then have the members, divided into small groups, act out those that are most meaningful to them.

Sue Jennings (1973) has used group members to photograph their group engaged in a variety of creative exercises, and has also brought in an outside photographer. She has found this particularly facilitative, especially in that it gives the leader a visual record of the whole group, and enables the members to be natural despite the camera, as they grow used to its presence.

PHOTOGRAPHS IN THE TREATMENT OF PEOPLE WITH EATING DISORDERS

Wessels makes excellent use of family photographs in treating people with eating disorders. His clinical material shows how the prevailing themes in anorexia are vividly illustrated in his patient's photographs. This patient was able to detect in her family album the childhood isolation, the lack of closeness in the family, and the repeated need to please her parents through being a 'good little girl'. Images of father are lacking, reflecting his absences. Where photographs with her mother are concerned, the patient:

> . . . describes her mother's connection with her as one of 'positioning' as opposed to touching and loving . . . She goes on to describe the photograph as 'lacking closeness, unnatural and posed,' which is a metaphor for her relationship with her mother.
>
> (Wessels 1985: 97)

Most importantly, the patient, who had been nicknamed 'lard bucket' as a child by her father, was able to see from her childhood photographs the image distortions that she had by now firmly internalised.

In addition, Wessels comments that his patient had not been able to identify or face these issues in any depth until they began to work with her album. He concludes that 'the visual nature of this technique lends itself well to working with a disorder that is highly concerned with appearance and body image'.

It would be unproductive, in my opinion, to focus solely on the physical aspects of an eating problem, and to work only with feelings about food and body-image. These need to be seen as symbolic of an underlying emotional problem, not as the root of the problem. Through working with photographs, and exploring distorted views of body-image, the patient may also see reflected there the other, emotional distortions she has absorbed.

Through using the camera, American therapist Linda Milligan endeavoured to counteract the obsessive and addictive behaviour which she perceived amongst her eating disorder patients. She saw that such behaviour interfered with their interpersonal skills, sense of play, creativity, self-awareness, self-esteem and body-image. She devised a project to help patients look at their bodies in less stressful way, at the same time giving them a chance to play and create. The task for the patients was to take pictures that incorporated the human form, with at least one full figure and one close up of some part of the body.

Patients worked together, to help them overcome the considerable anxiety, with the therapist giving much suppport. Not all could risk total exposure to the camera but all were willing to have some part of them photographed. Some would have only their faces taken, for others hands and feet were safe.

Most patients became playful, less perfectionistic, more creative and talkative as the session progressed. They became involved in decision-making as they set up images to photograph. This increased their problem-solving skills as well as their interpersonal skills. Learning to use the camera helped raise their self-esteem. For many patients, seeing the end result was exciting and they looked at the image of themselves in a less critical manner. For others, seeing the image of themselves was very difficult; some saw the weight they had gained and could not move away from the related anger. A few were able to go beyond their first reaction and become more self-accepting.

Some therapists use video feedback to help patients with eating disorders gain a more realistic image of self and body. McRea has used such methods with obese patients:

> . . . it appears that the achievement of a realistic body-image is therapeutically important for weight loss. While the obese devalue themselves, they will fail to attain a high self-regard, and this is one of the most significant factors in the battle to lose weight.
>
> (McRea 1983: 100)

Gottheil, Backup and Cornelison (1969) have used video to help combat denial in a case of anorexia nervosa. After several sessions of self-image confrontation, the patient at last began to change her image of herself, feeling that her thinness had become unattractive and disturbing.

LOSS AND BEREAVEMENT

Photographs are widely used in therapy with those who are grieving or preparing for some kind of loss. This may be related to death, divorce, or personal injury such as disfigurement or amputation.

In Canada, Judy Weiser is engaged in the use of photographs in therapy with AIDS patients. This kind of therapy will involve patients using photographs for the purposes of life review and also to help clarify personal values, to reflect on the self, and for personal construct work.

When the patient is mourning the loss of someone close, the photographs offers a means of enabling the dead person to be 'brought into' the therapy room. This symbolic and healing resurrection enables the agony of prolonged mourning to be mitigated, and helps the image of the dead person to be laid to rest within the inner world of the bereaved.

Unresolved grief may unconsciously wreak havoc for years after the actual death. It is often difficult to work through and express such grief freely, in a way that will enable the lost relationship to be finally ended. This process takes time. The photograph can magically provide this, making the dead person timelessly 'available', so that any unresolved feelings can therefore be explored 'with' that lost person.

It may also be useful to help a bereaved patient to look at photographs of other members of the family, for this will underline the fact that the person who has died is only one part of a support network which continues to exist although one member is lost. A video of a dead person is also especially moving because it can appear to bring that person to life again.[2]

Clinical illustration: Martin

Martin had been in therapy for about eight months when, of his own accord, he brought along his photograph album, a treasured collection of family pictures that he had assembled himself as a teenager.

He clasped it nervously, as he spoke about the dreadful headaches he was continuing to suffer and an addiction to work that left him feeling exhausted and drained. Martin's relationships with women tended to end leaving him feeling powerless, rejected and empty.

Twenty-two years ago, when he was 18, Martin's elder sister, Anna, had died, after a long illness. He had been very dependent on her, for she had always supported him and listened to his concerns in a family that repressed feelings.

After her death, Martin closed up emotionally, becoming the 'strong' one in the family, never showing his grief, or admitting it to himself. His sister's name was never mentioned in the family, and he had difficulty in saying her name himself. He had not looked at her photographs for years, finding them too overwhelmingly painful. The distance he created was a way of avoiding the conflicting ambivalent feelings that were bound up with the memory of his sister.

The fact that he was now bringing her pictures to therapy seemed to indicate a readiness to begin to face the depths of his grief. When he first came, Martin had no conscious awareness that his symptoms were in any way related to unresolved mourning. Through the work with photographs, he soon began to realise that his present feelings of emptiness at the end of relationships resonated with the losses of his past.

Martin looked afraid as he tentatively opened the album, and showed me a small black and white picture of Anna.

'This my sister, aged 18, on the beach. It is the last photograph that was taken of her.'

He glanced at the photograph, then looked away, towards the trees through my window. Outside, it was beginning to snow. For a while, we watched the first snowflakes drifting onto the bare branches. Soon, he was weeping softly. There were no words, but tears drenched his face. We sat together, sad and silent, aware of a beginning.

When he spoke, his voice was softer than I had ever heard it before: 'Taking out this photograph, it's like a way of saying that she's not forgotten. You see, I have blocked off all thoughts of her up to now. . . .'

'It was too painful to allow yourself to think about her. . . .' I said.

'Yes . . . I suppose I hoped that the feelings would all go away. I feel so guilty about that. . . .'

He looked at her photograph again, crying freely and addressing himself to me: 'I feel sorry that I made her so distant. . . .'

I ventured: 'I guess it might be hard to tell her that . . . but it may be important. . . .'

He looked at his sister, and began, for the first time in twenty-two years, to address her: 'I cut off because of all the pain, Anna.'

He buried his face in his hands and, for, several minutes, his body was racked with sobs. The huge intensity of his pain pervaded the room, and we stayed with the enormity of it all, with the confusion, torment and desolation of his grief. This felt new, repressed and unexpressed until that time.

As his anguished cries subsided a little, Martin looked again at his sister's photograph.

He stared at it, in silence, for a long, long time.

He told her: 'I love you . . . I have never forgotten you . . . I am sorry.'

Over the ensuing weeks, as we worked on with his album, Martin was also able to get in touch with some anger with his sister for leaving him; he had up till then avoided facing the anxiety engendered by such conflicting feelings. He had much grief to work through, for Martin was not yet ready to leave her or say goodbye. He was trapped in a wish to look for her, and a fear of finding her.

Gradually, in his everyday life, Martin felt that he was becoming more in touch with his feelings and less afraid to face his photographs. Weeks later, he was able to tell me: 'At first I feared the album. Now it's friendly.'

But he still felt Anna had drifted away from him each time he opened his album. It was risky to face the mixture of feelings that were triggered by the memory and the sight of her.

As he risked speaking to her picture, Martin was addressing an internal image of his sister:

'I want you with me . . . why did you go? Why did you have to leave me, Anna?' he sobbed, 'I've looked for you. I look for you in women, now. I look for you, Anna, everywhere.'

Silence. I asked what was happening for him. He did not answer. Then: 'She has not left me . . . she is still here. She is telling me so now. . . . She was always there to talk to me, you know, because she was ill, she was always there. And then, suddenly, she wasn't. I feel that desperate loneliness, now, just like when she died. But I could never show it, I never have shown it.'

Martin looked again at the photograph for ages. It felt as though he was attempting to absorb it, to take into himself the lost image of his lost sister; perhaps also he was wanting to compensate for the years of not looking at it or acknowledging it.

Martin's headaches began to lessen, and he stopped working so frantically. Each time, in the session, as he opened the album at the same picture of Anna, he felt she had become distant again, and each time, as I encouraged him to speak to her, she grew nearer, and nearer.

As each session went by, it took less time for Anna to become close to him: 'I do not want you to go. . . . I feel guilty. . . . My guilt is not about before your death, but after. I tried to forget you. I have had such pain, Anna. My head has felt as though it would burst with the pain.'

He was now linking the physical pain with the emotional: 'But I can't have you with me . . . I can't picture you without the photograph yet. I don't want you to go. . . .'

After this, he began to carry the small picture of Anna around with him constantly, as if to absorb the image through keeping it close.

Gradually, as the weeks and months passed, he was able to bring the album to therapy, without feeling the need to open it, and then to leave it at home and still be able to keep the memory of Anna with him.

He was at last able to talk freely, and sometimes joyfully, about past times with his sister, for he had internalised her image and, through working with her photographs, had finally let go of the pain and grief he had so long repressed. The album no longer represented a collection of painful and difficult memories; he had reframed it, and there was now no need to avoid it or cling to it.

The photograph as a 'linking object'

The photograph of Martin's sister was a way of connecting himself to her. However, this photograph also functioned to trap the emotions in a kind of stasis, a time-freeze. Through using it therapeutically, Martin was able to focus on the process of mourning, to release the store of feelings and to find relief and resolution.

Vamik Volkan describes the photograph used in this way as a 'linking object':

> These are objects typically treasured by people unable to resolve their grief – something that magically provides the illusion of communication with the dead. The pathological mourner can control this illusory communication, turning it on by musing over the object and turning it off by putting the object out of sight in an accessible place. Thus he can either recall the dead person or reject (kill) him in a pattern that reflects the ambivalent relationship of the past. The heavy emotional investment the mourner makes in such an object makes it a key with which to unlock the emotionality that then becomes manageable and even healing when the reasons for the previous failure to grieve are identified and both the emotionality experienced and the interpretations that accompany it are brought under the scrutiny of the patient's observing ego.
>
> (Volkan *et al.* 1976: 179)

It will also be seen in the following pages that photographs were used as transitional objects by the doomed children of the Holocaust, whose parents gave them family photographs before they were taken away.

THE USE OF PHOTOGRAPHS IN THERAPY WITH SURVIVORS OF TRAUMATIC EXPERIENCES

When people have had very traumatic experiences, when they have been tortured, abused, imprisoned, attacked or have been victims of war or disaster, there may, naturally, be a wish to forget. Photographs of, or reminiscent of, past traumas may precipitate depression and resurrect pain and guilt. They must, therefore, be used with care.

There are survivors who do not want to tell their stories or to look at photographs from the past. They need to relegate the pain to the depths of their unconscious and use all available defences to repress the memories, stifle the images. These defences have a definite protective function and need to be firmly respected. The photographs, often grim reminders of desperate past experiences, assault and wound their senses. For such people, the visual confrontation with a pain too great to bear is an abuse. They have been too disturbed to look; the photographs represent an unwanted intrusion into their lives.

But such is the nature of the human mind that, for many people, traumatic memories cannot be put to rest merely because the conscious mind wills it; they haunt survivors throughout their lives, manifesting themselves in many ways, such as fearful nightmares and flashbacks.

Photographs, whilst awakening the most painful of memories, can also help to heal the traumatised survivor, through enabling the past to be reworked in a therapeutic way.

The silent witness: the Holocaust photograph

There are in existence many photographs of the Holocaust; whilst most of these were taken by the Nazis, for official purposes and identification of concentration camp inmates, a smaller collection was taken by the victims themselves, the resistance and by Jewish underground photographers. Often carrying hidden cameras, they risked death if discovered.

For decades, these photographs have survived against the odds to tell their solemn stories; stories of suffering upon suffering, faded hopes, forgotten dreams, thwarted ambitions. They speak of pain, humiliation and death. For many victims and witnesses of the Holocaust, the photographs represented some kind of hope; if the people must die, then at least the photographs would survive. Buried, smuggled, hidden, sent abroad, treasured above all other possessions, grimly clung to despite threats of dire punishment, the photographs gave some comfort to the sufferers.

Now, years later, such photographs are used therapeutically by survivors in a general way, or they may be brought into the therapy situation.

The personal therapeutic use of Holocaust photographs

In their personal lives, these photographs allow the survivors to tell their stories and in some way to work through their traumas; they also provide evidence and confirmation of a grim past. Survivors instinctively and sometimes unconsciously employ photographs in their intrinsic desire for self-healing. Often alone with their pictures, they engage in repeated looking, and memories flood, tears are shed.

Some indicate that the very possession, the *having* of the photographs, brings healing. One survivor hardly ever had to look at the photograph of his lost brother; he just knew it was *there* and that knowledge brought some peace. The personal photographs of family and friends lost in the Holocaust still provoke tears, pain, longing. Almost without exception, these photographs have powerful effects on surviving relatives.

For Holocaust survivors do not have the usual aids to grieving that are available to most bereaved relatives; there are no tombstones, no grave-yards. They had no funerals, symbols or rituals to help them move steadily through their grief. So, often, their mourning remains undone, arrested. For many, photographs are the only external trace of the dead. They remain as a potent way to work through the grieving process, which will still inevitably be protracted and incomplete.

Holocaust photographs in therapy

Some survivors, having formal therapy, will sometimes bring photographs to use with their therapist, whether in a group or individual setting.[3]

Such photographs can enable some kind of understanding and working through of traumatic experiences; they can provide a therapeutic bridge between the generations, also helping the children of survivors to under-stand and make some kind of sense of their parents' experiences and to use this knowledge in some productive way for the future.

Issues of understanding and insight are central to any therapeutic endeavour; one survivor, who spent the first three years of his life in Bergen Belsen, gained insight into himself and his own history through contemplating his adult attitudes to horrific concentration camp photographs:

> I recognised the heaps of dead bodies in the photographs, but I did not experience the expected feelings of horror, as others do. I thought I had no response, that I was blocking my feelings. Then I realised – my response was *to the familiar*. These scenes were everyday ones for me – I played amongst dead bodies for the first three years of my life.

A most important function of the Holocaust photograph in therapy is to help the survivor to put fragmented remnants of memory into some kind of context, to give give them chronology. In enabling continuity, the photographs permit the start of reconstruction and recreation. The need is to rekindle the past in a manner that will help survivors come to terms with it, so that they can mourn and lay the ghosts:

> Their greatest need is the need to recount the experience in a meaning-ful, integrated sequence so the past can be reviewed as if it were more ordinary than it was. The constant barrage of seemingly nonsensical fragments of recall are extremely disturbing until placed in context. In this way, even the worst memories can at least be examined with the

benefit of greater understanding. . . . Survivors who present for care generally have an intense desire to relate to their life story but not through associative and interpretive methods. A need exists to reconstruct a chronological sequence of their experience in which to fit the repetitive or intrusive memories.

(Krell 1990: 19)

As we have seen in Chapter 2, photographs provide an excellent medium through which to enable such vital reconstruction, to create a cohesive whole out of chaos and confusion.

They also facilitate a sharing of the past with an empathic other, offering visual evidence of the most inconceivable experiences: 'The sights I have just seen are so unbelievable that I don't think I'll believe them myself until I've seen the photographs.'[4] These are the words of Margaret Bourke-White, sent by *Life* magazine to photograph Buchenwald after its liberation in April 1945. (The allies at this time hoped that publication of photographs from the camps would re-educate the population and shock them into realising the truth about the Nazi regime.)

The photographs were needed as confirmation, as evidence, of what the photographer herself had seen and knew to be true. The repeated looking, the fixing of the horrendous images on paper, rendered the experience believable, even to the photographer. Memory itself felt suspect because of the extreme nature of the spectacle. This phenomenon, of being uncertain or doubting about the reality of a terrible experience in the past, is common to most survivors of traumatic stress.

Photographs and the survivors of the Hillsborough disaster

For survivors of the Hillsborough football disaster, photographs have provided a way of confirming the terrible events of 15 April 1989. The reconstruction of the Hillsborough crowd from photographs and videos has enabled survivors – and their helpers – to gain a sense of continuity as well as being evidential to the police. Such pictures help with the syndrome of post-traumatic stress, a feature of which is loss of memory and awareness about the traumatic event, because of shock and bewilderment.

Like photographs of the Holocaust, these Hillsborough pictures have been used both as a general therapeutic aid, and in the therapy situation. One survivor carried a picture of himself at the scene which was on the front page of the *Daily Mirror*, 'to convince myself I was there – to reassure myself that I was not dreaming it'.

The use of Hillsborough photographs as an adjunct to counselling

Social workers at the Hillsborough centre in Liverpool offered clients the options of using the photographs and newspaper cuttings, and also videos of Hillsborough, in conjunction with counselling. For some, these were invaluable in helping work through their recent trauma.

One survivor was especially troubled because he was unable to remember much about his ordeal. A video showed that, for a whole thirty minutes, he had been physically trapped by corpses, causing him oxygen starvation. The man was unsure as to whether he had blacked out during that time, or whether he was blocking emotionally, but the video helped him to confirm exactly what had happened to him during the block in his recall.

For a survivor who had tried in vain to save his brother that day, photographs and videos helped him deal with survivor guilt and also allayed fears that he could have done more to save his brother's life. The pictures helped him to positively identify the enormous efforts he had made, and to reinforce the fact that he could not have done more to try to save his brother.

Photographs have therefore played a considerable role in the working through of post-traumatic stress symptoms caused by the disaster, enabling some kind of endorsement and verification of the survivors' terrifying experiences.

The therapeutic use of photographs with survivors of sexual abuse

Within the internal world of the sexually abused child, and of the adult abused as a child, are many, many horrific images, frozen snapshots of incidents that haunt and continue to abuse the mind. These are the pictures that were *not* taken, leaving the survivors terrifyingly isolated with their memories, bereft of external confirmation of their traumas. They are left to rely on the fragmented memories of childhood.

When these memories are corroborated by no one, and worse, when they are vociferously denied by others in the family, survivors can feel as though they are going insane, as if their experiences were not in line with real events and cannot be verified. Fear of punishment and of not being believed, self-doubt and shame may also prevent abuse survivors from sharing their terrible secrets.

Photographs of abusing families that do exist often look quite innocuous, for hiding feelings becomes a necessary part of survival for abused children; they become adept at putting on a face for the world – and for the camera. However, many photographs in the possession of survivors, though appearing innocent enough, can in fact provide startling revelations about the nature of the family's relationships. Often, these have not been looked at by the abused woman[5] for years, because of their ability to disturb, either consciously or unconsciously.

When patients experience the accepting atmosphere of therapy with a therapist who demonstrates belief, trust and empathy, they may, in time, remember and share some of the hidden pain of the past. Once the survivor has risked this sharing, she can perhaps be helped to find within her family photographs elements that will express much about the secrets in the family; these photographs can be used to considerable therapeutic effect. Let us now explore how such pictures may assist in some of the stages in the process of therapy with the incest survivor.

Photographs help to fill the gaps for people who may have blocked certain painful details of their past. Pamela had been in therapy for many months when she remembered that her father had sexually abused her. Only when she looked again at a photograph of him in a certain chair did she fully remember how her father abused her whilst sitting there; she had up to then always wondered why that particular photograph – and the sight of that chair – had made her feel so uncomfortable.

Sexually abused women enter therapy with feelings of enormous shame and guilt, often believing that they were responsible for the abuse, because they were in some way abnormal or that they seductively invited it and could have stopped it. Here photographs of the patient as a child can be invaluable in reminding her that she *was* a child – helpless, innocent and powerless against the strength of the abuser.

Hall and Lloyd (1989) use photographs in this way, and also contrast photographs of the child with those of the abuser, to emphasise in comparison the child's total physical inability to fend him off. This use of photographs helps to correct memory distortions about size and strength that will have kept the survivor locked into guilt.

One woman saw for herself that the child she had been when abused did not even have breasts; this realisation helped her to see the naivety, immaturity and innocence of the supposedly 'seductive' little girl, whom she had previously blamed and vilified.

Reaching the inner child[6]

Within the abused adult, there is a child who is in pain still, crying out for care and love. For so long, this child has wept inwardly, silently, and her tears have been unseen, her cries unheard. It is as if this inner child is buried within an oubliette, within the secret dungeon of her past, punitively forgotten.

And even now, instead of listening to her, the adult survivor, having internalised the image of her abusive parent and the derogatory messages about herself, further abuses the child within, pressurising her into believing she *was* bad. She will see the child within as a blameworthy, worthless creature, someone whom she despises.

She may even harm this image of herself, in acts of self-mutilation. Paradoxically, such acts may bring a kind of relief, for the abused person has learned that once a traumatic experience is over, there is some kind of brief relaxation. So, the abuse is recreated to dispel the terrible pain of fearful expectation. In addition, the abused woman is so used to having inappropriate anger and hate piled upon her, that she does the same to herself and cannot direct her rage outwards, towards the abuser, where it belongs.

The therapist will help the patient to reach her child within, so that she can learn to nurture and protect her in a way that she never experienced in childhood. The adult resources that the patient already has are strengthened so that, instead of repeating past patterns of hate and destruction towards the child within, the patient is empowered and encouraged to nurture her.

Photographs may be used here to help the patient communicate with her inner child. This connection may be difficult at first, because the patient has grown so used to having her child needs unheard and unmet, that she herself cannot hear the desperate inner voice from the past.

With care and understanding from the therapist, the patient can be asked to focus on a picture from childhood, to talk to the child that she was, to ask her how she feels, to reassure her that now she need no longer feel abandoned, afraid and alone. She can tell the child part of herself that the abuse was in no way her fault, and that she is not mad or bad. Thus, she provides a strong presence for that inner child, understanding and explaining in an adult way the confusion of feelings that the child experienced. Often, such patients carry around the photographs of themselves as children, so that they can help the inner child feel that there is now one strong, able adult to protect them from any abuse.

A significant absence of photographs

Hall and Lloyd make the point that

> . . . sometimes an incest survivor destroys photographs of herself and other family members. She may find the memories which are elicited by photographs too painful. If this is the case, the helper could ask the woman to obtain photographs from other family members.
>
> (Hall and Lloyd 1989: 169–70)

Where it is in no way possible to obtain photographs from childhood, then a snapshot of the inner child can be imagined and addressed within. Sometimes, the fact that an abused woman has no childhood photographs reflects the fact that she was not *seen*. When taking a photograph of someone, there has to be eye contact; perpetrators do not look into the eyes of their victims – that would make them too real, too human, instead of objects to be neglected and abused. Thus, some abused children are frequently neither seen nor photographed, for the importance of acknowledging and preserving their image is often immaterial within the abusing family.

Marcia had suffered a memory block between the ages of 2 and 12; as her memories returned in therapy, she realised that there were no photographs of her at all from this period of her life, although there were some taken before and after. It was during those ten years that she was being sexually abused by her father.

Some examples of photographs which reveal truths

In some cases, however, there are photographs of the abused child in her family that indicate all too readily what is happening within it.

Clare noticed that her grandfather, who abused her, had his arms firmly and possessively around her in all the photographs in which they appeared together. Stella saw that her father was looking at her in all family group photographs; she saw this as symbolic of her father's powerful obsessional feelings for his daughter. In Maria's album, she sees how physically close she and her father are, and that closeness brings back painful and disturbing memories about the emotional and physical hold her father had over her during her childhood. Delia cannot bear to look at pictures of her uncle's garden, where the abuse took place.

Vivienne brought to therapy a family photograph that showed herself as a child with her family, sunbathing in the garden (Photograph 23). At first, she did not feel that the photograph expressed anything about the interaction of the family but, on taking a closer look in therapy, she saw how that particular photograph said everything about the way her family related.

Aged about 16, Vivienne and her mother and younger brother are having their picture taken by father. We looked at Vivienne's posture and her expression. She appears ambivalent, wanting and not wanting to pose. Father has made her the centre of the photograph. Little brother is peripheral, to the right of the picture, half in shadow, whereas Vivienne is in the sun. Mother is on the left of the picture, and only part of her body is in the photograph, whereas her daughter is caught in her entirety. Mother has a smile on her face, but she leans back in her chair, with eyes closed, as she sunbathes. Vivienne says:

> This picture says it all. My father had me in his thrall, and though I hated and feared his attention, I was also mesmerised by him, deeply enmeshed in his powerful influence. I look somehow virginal here, yet I respond to his gaze with a seductive pose; this is what he wanted. You can see we have a secret together. I also look as if I am afraid, backing off, wary. My little brother is smiling broadly, trying hard to attract his attention. But it is all on me. I was special to him, too special, and I am trapped within that specialness. Mother smiles, yet sees nothing. This picture of her shows exactly what she was like – things were going on right in front of her. She saw, and yet she did not see; she just smiled sweetly, and prettily, to the world and pretended nothing was happening.

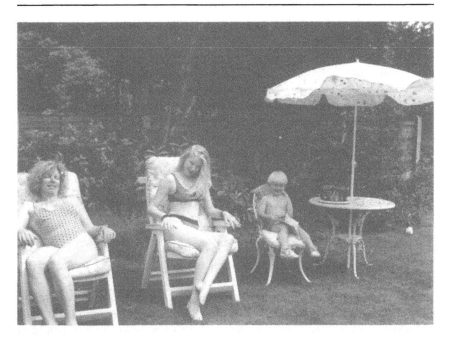

Photograph 23
Posed by models

The examples I have mentioned here were all instances where photographs helped to validate the survivors' experiences, enabling them to 'believe themselves' and trust their own perceptions – and their sanity.

The release of pent-up emotions: 'killing off' the abuser

Once the patient begins to realise that she is not to blame for the abuse, emotions begin to surface that have been repressed and turned inwards for years. Familiar photographs that may have seemed devoid of meaning begin to take on a whole new significance.

Photographs of herself as a child before the abuse enabled Nancy to get in touch with her anger at her abuser, for she saw the sweet, happy child she once had been, before her childhood had been spoiled. Her photographs graphically emphasised the contrast between this relaxed little girl and the child she was after the abuse. For then she became overweight and unhappy, alone, wary, with a detached, misty look in her eyes, hiding behind large glasses.

Within the safety of the therapy room, patients can learn to express anger at their abusers safely. Abused women have been conditioned to hold down their anger, and are often very afraid of their inner rage. Yet, within each abused adult is a scream so loud that it seems the earth would shatter were it released.

Often photographs are used to enable such powerful feelings to be expressed and discharged. They can be employed in an active way to disempower the abuser, with the patient destroying or mutilating the images. One therapist helped his patient burn photographs of her abuser, enabling a kind of freeing of the self from negative internalised images.

Such cathartic exercises, related to psychodrama, are most often followed by a sense of relief and a kind of celebration. In therapy groups for survivors of sexual abuse, life-sized dolls may also be used for the same purpose. Thus there is a combination of verbal therapy and more active therapy, a mix which addresses the inner and outer experiences of the abuse survivor.

Moving on: reorienting the self in the present

Just as photographs can help the survivor to get back into her child world, so they can be used to the opposite effect.

Hall and Lloyd (1989) use photographs in work with abused women to help bring regressed patients back to their adult state; after being regressed in therapy, the woman is shown photographs of her own, real-life child or of herself as an adult, which help to reorient her in the present.

Charlotte used photographs in therapy to emphasise the difference between past and present reality, not just in terms of herself, but also where her abusing father was concerned. She saw from his pictures how he had grown old and frail, looking quite unlike the terrifying monster she had experienced as a child. In contrast, photographs of Charlotte as an adult showed *her* tall and strong, empowered. Whilst she could not forget, she was able to move on and continue living her life more fully and courageously, knowing that the fears within her were old ones, and that she was now strong and her father weak.

Debbie saw the photographs of her parents 'change' only when she had given up on the hope that her parents would, one day, meet her needs, admit the abuse, make her better. She had given voice to her rage, feeling more power and energy. Up to this point, a large amount of energy had been used up in holding the anger down, leaving feelings of helplessness, depression and impotence.

Once the anger was expressed, however, Debbie held onto it, as if it were now the only way of connecting to her parents. She was still ambivalent about her feelings towards them, both reviling them and hoping for something from them.

It was the giving up of this fantasy, the letting go of the hope that her parents may, one day, change, that marked the beginning of real separation and individuation for Charlotte. It was at this point that, returning to photographs of her now elderly parents, the pictures were reframed, with her parents growing more real, shadows of those strong and feared figures from the past.

This process can give rise to feelings of loneliness, as if the survivor has been orphaned, for she has lost the fantasy of the parents she had hoped and longed for. In time, when the loss and the loneliness have been worked through, the incest survivor may be helped to create new, more hopeful and more healing images for the future.

Using photographs actively: Teresa's story

In order to attempt to make some sense of and work through her experience of sexual abuse by her father when she was a child, Teresa wanted to recreate some of her past feelings and experiences using the camera.

She made several collages, created out of old photographs, and also recreated some photographs which vividly showed how she felt as an abused child. As she was making these collages, cutting up the pictures and reassembling them to recreate her past experiences, she felt driven, as if this were something she had to do in order to express the pain and turmoil of her traumatic past:

> I did not have to think very hard. I just did it, cut up the pictures to fit in with my memories of the past. I had to do it. It all flowed. Afterwards I felt like it was all contained, there, within the collages, and that I had made many clear statements about my experiences that had been trapped within me. Because I was cutting things out, I was also making things clearer for myself. I think I was in some kind of altered state of consciousness. I felt I needed to reproduce how it actually was, how it was for me. The photographs helped me contain all my feelings.

Teresa portrays through her photographs the craziness of living in her family, the fear engendered by a mother strongly into spiritualism and who promised to haunt her forever: 'The family I was in was so crazy; I never understood what it was like to be on the outside. When I got outside, I was aware of everbody else's normality, and the craziness inside.'

Photograph 24 shows how Teresa portrayed herself and her feelings whilst she was being abused. Her photographs of abuse reconstruct those that were not taken. She is providing herself with much-needed visual images of her past, externalising the experiences, showing them to the outside world. In this picture, the mask she wears symbolises the feelings of dissociation that incest victims have. As Teresa remembers, and looks at the photograph she has created, she uses the present tense, as if it were happening to her in the here and now:

> I deafen myself, my ears go first – I can switch my whole physical body off. My face goes first when I'm under threat – my mother hit me round

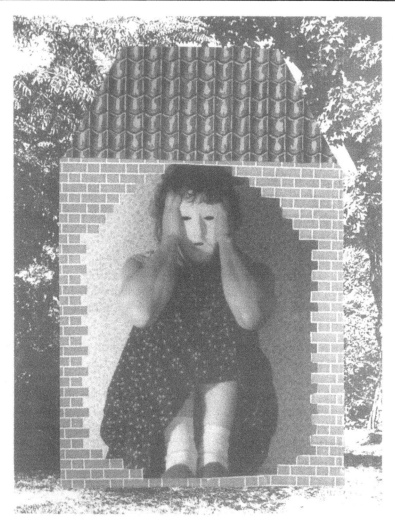

Photograph 24
Recreated photo

the head a lot. I sat like this in my bedroom as a child. I notice that there is a shadow on the left of me in the picture, and it is lighter on the right side. I feel that this symbolises the bad and good sides of me, or the going away, coming back aspects of me in this situation. I felt very cold when I was recreating this picture. I notice that I chose to wear skirts, and child-like shoes. I never wear skirts now.

I look very enclosed. When I made the picture, I did not know how it would turn out. I was feverish in the doing of it, and after it was

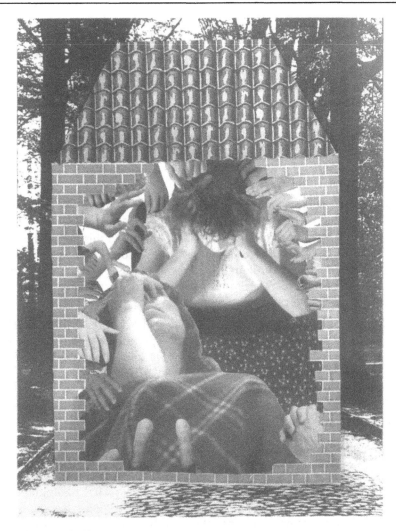

Photograph 25
Recreated photo

finished, I felt satisfied with it. It reminds me of Alice in Wonderland
– she did not fit – being either too big or too small.

The abused child's feelings of being a misfit are vividly expressed in this
photograph. She is treated like an adult in one way, and made to be very
big in terms of her role. Yet she also is small and insignificant, in that her
feelings are totally ignored.

In Photograph 25 Teresa has illustrated how it felt to know that she was
about to be abused again:

When father came up the stairs to my attic bedroom, I had feelings of panic, fearing that I wouldn't be able to get away inside myself and shut myself off from what was happening to me. That was the start of me panicking – I was working myself up to this while he was coming upstairs. A kind of feeling of falling forever, like a whirling figure of eight. That's what is expressed in the picture, and that is the kind of movement in the picture. The hands and fingers represent invasion. Look how still I am in it. In all the other pictures, as here, I am black and white all the time. I was unseen, invisible. They were the ones who were seen – and I show them in chaotic, mad colour, whirling around in an insane song and dance.

Teresa has used colour to express being seen, and also to express madness, chaos. Black and white symbolises invisibility in a mad world.

Recently, she tried to talk to her father, but found this impossible, and she began to cry. Father's response was to take out his wallet and show her that inside he kept three photographs of her as a child, which Teresa had never seen before. These photographs, and the place in which they were kept, had powerful symbolic meaning for Teresa:

I felt trapped when I saw them – it was as if I'd never grown up. They were to show me how important I still was to him; I felt that he had always wanted to take something of me, to keep a part of me for him, to extinguish something in me.

I was quite shocked that he had them, and at what I saw within those photographs. On one of them I looked very sensual, on another I looked very adult.

I feel that my childhood is trapped inside his wallet. . . . I *want* those pictures. My father has images of me that are trapped in his possession. These also perpetuate his story of being the loving father to me.

Teresa struggled long and hard with her own recreated photographs to work through some of her feelings about her past: 'It took me about a year to process these pictures, to work through the pain of what I saw within them. Now I do have some kind of resolution.'

Teresa's last collage shows how she has managed to reach the outside world, for it shows her as a freer, and happier adult. She uses her collection of photographic collages to go back again and again through her experiences, seeing new elements each time, and gradually working through her pain.

FROM PATIENTS TO THERAPISTS

It will now be evident that photographs have a considerable range of therapeutic uses, and I have in this chapter endeavoured to illustrate some of them. There are no doubt many more such areas to be explored that are beyond the scope of this book.

Having seen the many groups of people who can be helped through photographs, it is now time to alter the focus, and to take a close up of the therapist. For whatever the style of therapy, and whoever her patients are, the therapist is always faced with herself. Whether she is using photographs therapeutically with people who are old or young, black or white, male or female, she must struggle with her own personal values, constructs and self-image.

Unless the therapist has truly confronted her own reflections, both on a real and symbolic level, she cannot work with another person's images. At this point, therefore, we must consider in some detail the relationship between the photograph and the self.

Chapter 8

'Can it really be me?'
Photographs and the self

'Mr D. first sees his photograph three years after it was taken'

> Thank God I've shaved off the beard.
> That thicket of whitish-grey bristle!
> Can it really be me!
> I don't look like that now.
> I didn't look like that when I was young.
> I looked better when I was young.
> I looked younger when I was young!
> Remember the beautiful bone structure
> of that face? What have these jowls
> flanking that ridiculous goatee
> to do with me? You say
> I'm looking younger all the time
> but that's, isn't it, only because I've shaved.
> I used to be slim. I used to look forward
> to the future. That's why I grew
> and grew a beard, yes I am looking, yes,
> younger. Growing that beard
> was like making a sortie into No-man's Land
> to discover some features, some properties
> no one wishes to cultivate.
>
> (Mike Doyle, *Stonedancer*)

Throughout this book, I have stressed how important it is for therapists who use photographs to learn to know themselves through their own, personal photographs, in order to help their patients do the same. In this final chapter, I shall focus on how this task may be approached; I would hope to inspire readers of this book towards a journey of exploration that will mean that their photographs will never look the same again.

To begin, there will be a discussion of the wider context, of the panorama of stereotypical images within family and society that subtly influence us, colouring our picture of ourselves and others.

As the chapter develops, the focus will move inward, and there will be a close-up of people's responses to their own physical features, and an exposure of the associations, memories and feelings related to their appearance. This may prompt readers to contemplate their own self-images, and to learn to challenge any distortions or denial in the way the self is seen.

In order to know the self more clearly, an examination of the personal symbols and metaphors within photographs will follow; we shall also take a look at how the therapist may help the patient to understand the self through exploring personal photographic symbols. I shall, in addition, provide a selection of methods in which therapists may use photographs to further their understanding of self.

Examples will be given from both inside the therapy situation and outside, where photographs are used in a generally therapeutic way. The differences between these two kinds of photographic exploration are considerable; these were described in the Preface and must here be underlined. Therapists need, however, to have experienced, if at all possible, all kinds of ways of using photographs therapeutically, in order that they will have a firm foundation on which to build their skills in using photographs with patients. Maybe, as therapists, we can personally learn from the experiences of the patients in this chapter who have used their photographs to understand more about the self.

Therapists may share their photographs either with family and colleagues or perhaps they will take photographs into their own therapy. They may also wish to adapt some of these ideas to use with their patients in therapy.

LOOKING AT THE WIDER PICTURE: PUTTING THE SELF INTO CONTEXT

Photographs can be used to illustrate the influence of environment on the development of self-image. The way in which the media, for example, has visually portrayed women, disabled, homosexual and black people will have influenced the way we regard self and other. For example, photographic images of black people in negative roles, perhaps as prisoners or in demeaning jobs, are commonplace; there is an underlying, unconscious racism in this photographic selectivity. Sexist advertisements abound, with photographs showing women partially clothed or as dutiful, aproned housewives devoted to domesticity.

An examination of the photographs we have taken ourselves will further reveal aspects of how we view the world around us. How have we exposed our way of seeing through what have we chosen to photograph? What have we omitted?

Family photograph albums also reflect this social stereotyping, showing how strongly these attitudes have been absorbed into the individual and family psyche. Through our collections of photographs we may, therefore, begin to explore how powerfully and effectively our image of ourselves has been forged and shaped by various outside influences.

On the evidence of these preserved images of the past, we may consider whether we conformed to or were hampered by family and society's attitudes to the social, cultural, racial or sexual categories into which we were born. Such attitudes, compellingly restrictive, have persuaded many amongst us to live according to 'oughts' and 'shoulds', rather than to make our own rules. So often, we have been stereotyped, labelled, categorised, standardised, negated. Therapists need to peruse their own family album, to explore the constructions that may have been put on them during their developing years. They need to ask how they have been exhibited, portrayed, depicted, for the camera and within their immediate environment. Can they take those constructions apart, and find out who they really wanted to be?

How have our experiences affected *our* self-image? To what extent have these narrow ways of seeing limited us as therapists and restricted our responses to patients? As a therapist, if I am black, white, Jewish, Christian or agnostic, what difference does this make to my responses as a therapist?

Klaus's family album revealed photographs of his German family, with pictures of his father wearing Nazi uniform. Anxiously, and with considerable embarrassment, he apologised: 'I hope this doesn't offend you . . . I mean . . . being Jewish.'

From the earliest days of my childhood, I had grown to hate and fear the symbols of Nazism, and yet here they were, within the family album of my patient. Klaus was the same age as I, yet photographs of my father in the same era showed him wearing British army uniform; our families had been on opposite sides in a devastating war. Furthermore, my family photographs revealed a very different culture and reflected a context that could not have been more opposite to that of Klaus. Our contextual differences could never have been more starkly expressed than here, within these fading snapshots of the past.

Yet I was neither offended nor disturbed by the images of his father. There had developed by then a trusting therapeutic relationship, which worked both ways, so that the photographs were a means through which I could learn to understand – and accept – his context. As Klaus presented and explained this to me, I could quite easily see beneath any stereotyped images to the person within that uniform. They showed his father in a family setting, and were not just a pictures of a soldier onto which I could project my own assumptions and associations.

The photographs helped me, however, to increase my awareness of such issues. Actually *seeing* the images confronted me with my own feelings much more than verbal images could have done.

'This is the view from my window . . .': the house and the self

The image of the house often appears in dreams and, to many patients, it seems to symbolise the self and the body. In personal photographs, images of houses abound. They provoke deep emotions, intense and vivid associations, and may come to represent a whole set of feelings.

Pictures of one's childhood house can also stimulate a consideration of the kind of view one had of the world from within those familiar walls on both a real and a symbolic level. Patients sometimes take such pictures of their houses, past and present, into therapy. They are bringing the outside in, and giving the message – 'This is my context, this is where it has all happened.'

Gemma spotted for the first time symbolic similarities in photographs of her own perfectly maintained house and the house of her childhood, which had been obsessively managed by her strict mother. She also began to understand, as we perused the photographs that, like her mother, she had become a slave to the environment she herself had created. It had grown into a representation of a kind of inner monster, that threatened to devour her with its need for perfection and toil. She felt controlled by her relationship with her environment, just as she had, as a child, felt controlled by parental strictures.

Marianne showed me pictures of the grand, mansion house of her childhood, telling me how she had lived, fearfully, in an atmosphere of museum-like coldness. She was also revealing something of her culture, her context, the backcloth to her childhood world. This was a world of back and front stairs, acres of garden and staff quarters.

I found that, internally, I as therapist was comparing the photographs of this childhood house to my own, reflecting how the contrasts might mirror those in our life experience and in our very selves. What did the differences in our personal images symbolise about us as separate individuals in the world, and as therapist and patient? Could I relate to her difference and she to mine? Could I see the world through the 'windows of her house', or was I too restricted by my own frames?

How wide was the gap between us, signified by the difference in our images of the past? Could these differences be usefully acknowledged, or would they inhibit and restrict? How limited have I been by the environmental images that surrounded me?

Sex-role stereotyping

Therapists need also to explore the sex-role stereotyping that may have occurred within their own lives. If they are unaware of such issues, they will fail to help their patients understand how they have been unconsciously conditioned into adopting certain roles.

Hafner believes that fixed sex-role stereotyping lies at the heart of many marital difficulties and of much mental illness in marriage. These rigid ways of seeing self and other trap and restrict couples, hampering their individual growth and limiting their ability to relate healthily. Hafner explains the manifestations of such sex-role stereotyping:

> Women's maternal and nurturing roles are other attributes that are widely seen in stereotyped terms. Idealized mothers are generally regarded as patient, self-sacrificing, warm, affectionate, and responsive to the emotional needs of their children and others. They are not aggressive or overtly assertive, are guided by intuition and emotion rather than logic, and depend on their husbands for advice, guidance, and protection in areas beyond the domestic. They are altruistic and live for and through their children and husbands.
>
> In contrast, idealized fathers are seen as adventurous, competitive, and assertive, as well as aggressive if this is required to protect their own or their family's interests. They are ruled by logic rather than emotion and are required to suppress or deny feelings of weakness, helplessness, and timidity. They avoid the overt display of emotions indicating a distressed, sad, or fearful state. The expression of tender, loving feelings is not required of them, and they are not expected to be sensitive to the emotional needs of others or to publicly reveal their own personal worries, fears and doubts.
>
> (Hafner 1986: 16–17)

Photographs perpetuate sex-role stereotyping because they record and preserve it; however, paradoxically, they also make such behaviour available for examination, with a view to an intense reassessment of such long-held attitudes, bringing them into consciousness. Otherwise, they may pervade the whole of a person's life. If we look carefully, we may discover examples of such unconscious stereotyping of the sexes within our family albums and, of course, in those of our patients.

Photographic evidence of such conditioning is somewhat less apparent today, but it is still to be found in the albums of older people. It is visually indicated in terms of selected activities, dress and parental choice of toys.

Conforming to a desired cultural image

Photograph albums are full of people attempting to fit in with external images. It is important for therapists to discover how much they, too, hamper themselves by such restrictions, perhaps even conforming to a desired image of how a therapist 'should be'.

Maggie, previously introduced in Chapter 4, saw that as a child she had become adapted to the needs of the adults around her and linked this with a tendency to be over-apologetic as an adult.

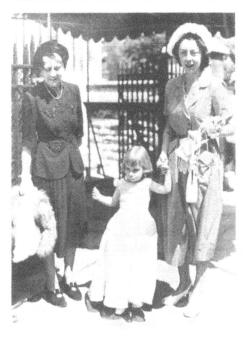

Photograph 26
© Maggie Wilson

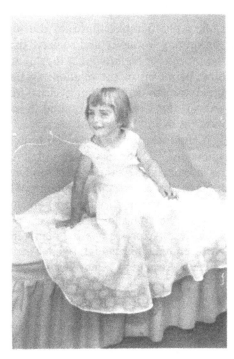

Photograph 27
© Maggie Wilson

Often, therapists who have had such an upbringing may find it difficult to confront their patients, or they may take on responsibility for their patients' problems.

Maggie had two childhood pictures which showed how she was becoming trained and submissive, losing her naturalness. In the first, Photograph 26, we see her as a bridesmaid. Maggie remembers that she had found the church dark and frightening. She looks quite uncomfortable, and it is interesting to note the way she is being held – with her arm up in the air. She felt defiant, refusing to smile for the photographer.

In the next picture (Photograph 27), however, Maggie notices that she is smiling and posing.

She reflects in her study:

> Suffice it here to say that the experience of being a bridesmaid was a profound one that has influenced my thinking and female ideology.
>
> What really lies below these photographs? At first, I appear sullen and will not look at the male photographer. Whereas a few weeks later, in a more relaxed setting, I conform to being the 'ideal' object of the male gaze. I have learnt how to conform.
>
> (Wilson 1991: 25)

From conformity to self-acceptance: the use of photographs as a measure of change in the self

Colin's photographs illustrate the high personal price that he paid for conforming to family and society; they also clearly document changes in the process of his lifelong struggle. As therapists we may learn from this how, by means of the relationship between the photograph and the self, there can be a confirming visual record of an individual's emotional growth. For Colin, this resulted in increased insight, strength and clarity in terms of self-image and identity.

A homosexual man in his late forties, Colin has fought within himself for autonomy, for freedom from an internal and external pressure to suppress his individuality. As the conflict resolves over the years of his life, his pictures begin to illustrate a new acceptance of his true identity and sexuality. Colin's photographs have also helped him understand and measure the stages of development in his life and have assisted him with chronology and memory.

Selected pictures graphically pinpoint the stages in his development from an uncertain, timid child, through a confused adolescence and into adulthood, where he eventually achieved some serenity and inner acceptance of himself.

A snapshot from childhood

In Photograph 28 we see Colin as a small child. The picture sums up some of the confusion that Colin must have experienced from an early age.

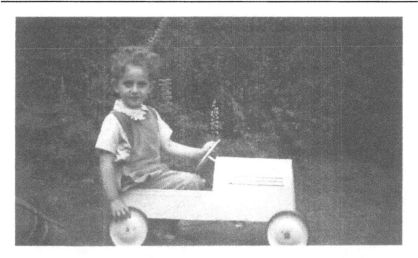

Photograph 28

There is considerable sexual ambiguity here, for he looks quite feminine. He is, at the same time, in a car, which was seen largely as a male symbol.

Colin felt that life would have been better had he been a girl. There was no emotional closeness with father, who he felt adored his sisters. Colin wonders if the fact he is gay is partly to do with this lack of fatherly affection – from childhood he has longed for someone male to love. He remembers:

> When my sister and I were young, father bought me a Meccano set and my sister a dolls' house. I wanted the dolls' house. I was often dressed in the same hand-knitted jumpers as my sister; they each had the same characters on – Wuf, Tuf and Muf.

We may wonder: why was he presented in this girlish way? As the only boy in the family, was it hard for the adults to recognise and confirm his maleness? Has this anything to do with his homosexuality?

Colin realised he was gay when he was eleven. This is his first clear memory, though he is aware there must have been earlier feelings. He hid his realisation from his family, for he felt his feelings were wrong and abnormal. He did not fit in with his family's image of him, and this made him feel bad and inadequate.

A painful, shameful adolescence

Colin looks at a photograph of his bar mitzvah, the ceremony at the age of 13, which marks and celebrates a Jewish boy's transition into manhood

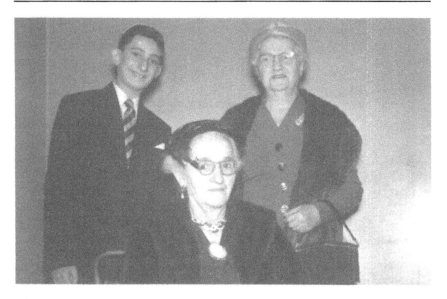

Photograph 29

(Photograph 29). He reflects that adolescence was a very difficult time for him: 'A cruel thing happened when I was adolescent. My looks changed, and I had sticky-out ears, and a big nose. I had an obsession that everyone in the family was good-looking except me.'

To compound all this, Colin was having difficulty with his sexual identity. His feelings of discomfort about his physical self were linked to these issues. He felt very different, physically inferior to his peers. At this time he was uncomfortable with photographs where he felt he 'looked effeminate in terms of body language, clothes, posture, hairstyle – I felt I was meeting neither my own nor others' expectations. At 13, I felt I was an ugly duckling. I avoided having pictures taken after that. I really suffered during that time, people called me hurtful names.'

Such shame and embarrassment about one's self may especially occur in adolescence, a very vulnerable time. To be photographed when one is feeling so self-conscious about one's appearance is excruciatingly painful, and Colin remembers such distress, and sees it reflected in his photographs. His shame, in relation to his looks and his emerging sexuality, was in fact experienced in response to being *looked at*, a fear of being seen by others:

> We often say that the shy man is 'embarrassed by his own body.' Actually this expression is incorrect; I cannot be embarrassed by my own body as I exist it. It is my body for the Other which may embarrass me.
> (Sartre 1957: 353)

Thus, from age 13 to 19, there is an absence of photographs. Colin realises that his shame prompted him thereafter to hide from the camera's all-seeing, all-recording, all-mocking eye. For the camera represents not only the other, the photographer, but a whole host of future others who threaten to gaze at its shaming work.

Here it must be emphasised that photographs are often absent during difficult sections of time in a person's life; we generally photograph the brighter side.

And so to adulthood . . .

At 19, Colin decided to have plastic surgery on his nose and ears. He was convinced that the operations would change his life. He was attempting to transform himself, externally, into the stereotyped image of the hetero-sexual man. He even tried to change his internal self by having aversion therapy. Photographs of this time show the differences in his appearance, which reflect his desperate wish to live up to family and social expectations.

Then there are pictures of his wedding, at age 27, and several photo-graphs taken during his ten-year marriage. During this time, Colin was constantly fighting against his true sexuality, pretending to the world. There are many photographs of this period of his life, showing him apparently happy. But, as he peruses these, Colin remembers that behind the smiles in the photographs he felt guilty, despite a happy act. He sees that this is a family pattern, reflecting also a similarity between him and his mother, in that she, too, was living a lie in an unhappy marriage. Father was also caught up in this need to live up to an image. Colin married because it was expected of him by family and society – 'After all,' he says, 'I was 27 and Jewish!'

Ten years on, Colin acknowledged who he was. The marriage ended soon afterwards. His life took on a different meaning as he began to question and re-evaluate; he changed career, becoming a bridge teacher.

This change is vividly shown in his photographs, where he begins to be himself, looking happier. This contrasts with the earlier photographs, where he was pretending to be happy – there is a greater abandon in the later ones, a freedom to be himself.

New insight . . .

Looking at his photographs also triggered a new awareness in Colin of how much he has always wanted to dress up. So many of the photographs show him wearing fancy dress at parties. Colin enjoys being in the limelight, for this feels very different to the obscurity of his childhood. He observes through his photographs, however, how the dressing up has changed:

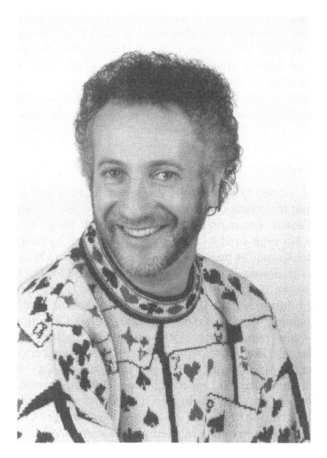

Photograph 30

Before I came out I did not feel OK about the dressing up – and the photos do reveal this discomfort. The motivation was largely sexual, because I had no other outlet for those feelings, which were inadmissible. I can now admit to them, so there is no need to channel them into dressing up. This links also with dressing in mother's clothes as a child, partly in the hope of being more accepted as a woman because life seemed better for women in our family.

Colin's dressing up now is about really enjoying the creative challenge, expressing and integrating all the selves within him, enjoying being centre stage.

Colin feels that Photograph 30 shows how far he has come – for he is happy with himself and the way he looks. There is a sense of fun about him now, and a firm feeling of identity expressed through the 'bridge' jumper. He seems to be saying, clearly, 'This is me.' Colin feels that he has now learnt to combine strength with creativity and that the picture symbolises this.

The photograph signifies Colin's redefinition of himself, a process that can be traced through his album. It is very different from his image within his family during his earlier years, when he felt unhappy, and labelled as weak and weedy.

It may be a helpful exercise to consider how one would like one's photographic history to be changed. As Colin pondered on his photographic life-story, he added that if he could reconstruct his childhood through photographs, he would wish to recreate a child who was not afraid of playing football, a child who fitted in with others, and who did not feel so much the odd one out in his family.

DISCOVERING THE 'I' THROUGH THE 'EYE' OF THE CAMERA

Therapists need to become sensitive to their own images, and to their feelings about these. Those having therapy themselves may find it helpful to bring photographs into their own therapy.

As therapists, exploring pictures of ourselves through life, in the way that Colin has done, we also may search for parts of the self that are disliked, reviled, hidden. The external, physical aspects of ourselves reflect the internal, therefore, we may discover much about our inner world in this journey through our photographic images.

During this process of self-examination through photographs, this retrospective view of our life, we may start with pictures of childhood, describing the child that we were, noting carefully the adjectives that are used in this description. They will be meaningful, for they will reveal attitudes towards the inner child aspect within the adult self. For example, I have heard patients in therapy variously describe their 'child' in a photograph as 'naughty', 'big-headed', 'stupid' or 'ugly'. I have endeavoured to help such patients to reframe the concept of self through gaining an understanding of what lies behind the unthinking label they have given themselves.

As we move on to pictures of the adult self, we may ask what aspects of ourselves we have not wanted to see and have chosen to *overlook*. Attitudes to our own body will be revealed in the way we pose for the camera, perhaps holding in our stomach, or lifting the head to hide a double chin, disguising facial lines by smiling only slightly. Perhaps we have a 'good' side and a 'bad' side, or attempt to project an image for the camera and the world – one that is kindly, or assertive, intelligent, cheerful perhaps, or studiously serious. In doing this, parts of the self are being denied. We may, in addition, take note of any differences over the years in the way we see ourselves, and also observe our feelings about the inevitable changes in our faces and bodies.

Our facial images are especially important to all of us. Most of us want to have photographs of ourselves; when we are presented with a group photograph, the majority of us scan the picture quickly to look for our own face first. When the daguerreotype was first invented, it was principally used to take pictures of faces. People wanted to record their image for posterity, to give themselves some kind of *individual* recognition and importance in the world, to capture their essence forever.

Many times, however, a photograph is discarded because it is 'no good'. The reflection it offers us comes as a shock, and sometimes people deny the picture is of them. Perhaps this is because it does not fit the ideal, internalised image of the self. Milgram describes some reactions to pictures of self from the earliest days of photography:

> If you had never had a photograph taken of yourself, the best clue to what it would look like was based on what you had seen in a mirror. And that is where the surprise came in. For individuals almost never reject what they see in the mirror, but hundreds of Daguerreotypes were angrily denounced by men and women who knew they were more comely than the photograph showed. What they should have learned is that the psychological preparations made before looking into a mirror are such that we do not affront our own self-image. Even today, individuals are constantly rejecting unflattering snapshots, firmly believing that they could never look as bad as the photograph showed. But such reactions rarely come upon looking into a mirror. Perhaps the old 'a mirror offers us a thousand faces; we only accept one,' contains the relevant wisdom. The camera, by freezing our faces at a particular moment, from a particular viewpoint, often gives us one of those faces that we would prefer not to accept.
>
> (Milgram 1977: 341)

So, consider: what is a 'good' photograph? One that puts us in a good light? If that is so, what on earth does it *mean*? I have heard people say of a 'bad' photograph: 'It doesn't flatter me at all.' Do we have to get the camera to flatter us? These and other questions may emerge as we consider our photographic histories.

It is most important to examine the 'rejects', the snaps that we hide, alter, censor, tear up, discard. We will then learn to challenge any rigidities in the way we view ourselves. It is only when, as therapists, we have taken on board these disowned images of ourselves, that we will be able to help others accept their whole picture of self, 'warts and all'. In order to know more about ourselves, we must also be willing to risk being seen, and perhaps photographed, in all our aspects, to confront the ideal image to which we may cling.

Family resemblances

Robert, aged 16, closely resembles his great-grandfather, especially in one particular photograph:

> People say he looks like me. Even my best friend looked at the photo and asked 'What were you dressed up like that for?'
>
> Sometimes it's hard to feel that it is a different person from me in the photograph. I have heard that he wasn't very nice, he was a difficult person. I wish I didn't know that. The fact that someone could look so like me and not be someone people could get on with. . . . I don't like it.
>
> The picture has always represented to me the bad side of me. . . . I'm not sure what that is. I put it face down sometimes. And there is a look in the picture, it's not very soft, it's stern, cold. . . . (He ponders on the photograph for several minutes.)
>
> It's *not* me. I'm not like that. I don't feel like that. Seeing the picture is like seeing an empty shell of me, without me in it. It's very confusing, though; there's an eeriness that we never knew each other and yet there's a strong link between us because we look so alike.

Studying photographs of the self is a complicated matter, for we inevitably see many reflections within our own face. Evidence of our past experience, of the pain and the joy in our lives, is irrevocably etched upon our features. Furthermore, like Robert, we will catch glimpses of relatives, even discovering ancestral likenesses that stretch back towards the roots of our family tree. Each individual is therefore a unique and composite blend of experience and ancestry.

As we turn the pages of our album, and recognise similarities in noses, eyes, foreheads, mouths, face shape, hair colour, build, we may wonder: 'How does it really feel, personally, to resemble another person?' It is important to identify our projections onto someone in a photograph, so that we may be able to differentiate ourselves from others and know ourselves as individuals.

If we have admired these people we resemble, or heard positive stories of them, we may need to live up to their image; this may be either inspirational or constraining.

On the other hand, as with Robert, if we bear a likeness to someone who is reputedly nasty, or whom we have actually feared or hated in childhood, it can be an enormous burden to see ourselves wearing an approximation of that person's face.

Disturbing questions may then emerge:

'How else am I like him?'
'How much am I like him?'
'Can I come to terms with the possibility that, as well as sharing his physical features, I may also share aspects of his personality?'
'If he has been abusive, what about the "abuser" in me?'

If we deny a family resemblance, are we afraid to ask such difficult questions of ourselves?

Changing the image: separation and individuation

Consider the statement 'You look just like your mother.' On hearing this, you may wonder exactly what it *means*. It may feel like a compliment, or it may produce uncomfortable questions in your mind, doubts, qualms, uncertainties. What aspects of yourself and the other do you immediately think of when someone spots a photographic resemblance?

Whom do you see when you look at pictures of mother – or father? How do you react to photographs of each parent at your age? What are the similarities and differences?

For some of us, it is hard to accept any similarities, and to realise that we may have inherited parts of a parent, for better or worse. For instance, if we are struggling to separate, striving for independence, then physical resemblances to either parent may painfully underline our ambivalent connection with them. If, however, we have managed to individuate, then the physical similarities will feel comfortable, for we will have integrated them as autonomous individuals.

If aspects of your parents continue to live on in you, can you identify these? Maybe there are parts of them that you have rejected, allowed to die, and parts you wish to keep.

> 'Why, you look just like your mother!' a woman said to me recently. I thought she meant I was wearing my mother's tight, anxious look. But she was thinking of something else. 'The last time I saw her,' this woman went on, 'your mother bid a grand slam. It was four o'clock in the morning, and she made it!'
>
> Stories of my mother's courage have always excited me. The photos of her I love so much hang over my desk – jumping a horse over a high brick wall, wearing a daring two-piece bathing suit twenty-five years ago when she was my age. Why have I refused to credit her for the abilities and emotions I have tried to incorporate in myself?
>
> (Friday 1983: 459)

Only through coming to terms with the reality of her mother, was Nancy Friday able to really *see* her. Once she had stopped hoping for an ideal mother image and had divested her of the role of the fantasy mother for whom she had longed, she was able to see the real value of her mother, and the positive aspects that she had inherited.

At times, it is difficult to see images of parents as real, whole people, to let them be fully rounded human beings. Can we see our parents clearly, or are their images clouded with our projections? Have we invented the kind of ideal parental images we would want, so that our parents' photographs are shrouded in illusion, in wishful thinking? Are we able to see our parents as whole people, or are they partial figures, representations of disowned aspects of self?

If there is still a need to invent the kinds of parent we would have wished for, then it will not be possible to see a clear picture. We will remain fixed, connected by fantasy to an unreal image.

The photograph reflects back our projections, our psychological inventions, in a way that may make us question them; we may then experience the clarity – and the disillusionment – of real seeing. If, as therapists, we have not learned to identify our own fictions and fabrications, how can we help patients to do so? It is only when such illusions are challenged and dispelled that real individuation and separation can occur.

Photograph and symbol

In using the photograph as an aid to self-discovery, and in order to help the patient become more adept at discovering the self in therapy, much attention must be given to symbolism. Let us now explore the meaning of this term in relation to the photograph, discovering how photographic images become symbols.

We invest various images in our photographs with extended meanings that come from our inner world, thus creating visual symbols:

> an image is symbolic when it implies something more than its obvious and immediate meaning. It has a wider 'unconscious' aspect that is never precisely defined or fully explained. Nor can one hope to define or explain it. As the mind explores the symbol, it is led to ideas that lie beyond the grasp of reason.
>
> (Jung 1978: 4)

Where photographs are concerned, the experience that Jung describes above can be a powerful one; looking at the photograph may revivify repressed symbols and provide strikingly potent material for recollection and association.

We may have taken such photographs ourselves and, consciously or unconsciously, have created various meaningful symbols in so doing. Alternatively, we may have selected various old photographs, taken by others in the past, to represent aspects of our inner world, past and present. In both cases, the photographs may be rich in symbolic meaning and they may become very important to us in terms of externalising inner visions.

People use symbols as a way of representing aspects of their experience of the world, both inner and outer. Our environment is rich in material from which we can make symbols:

The history of symbolism shows that everything can assume symbolic significance: natural objects (like stones, plants, animals, men, mountains and valleys, sun and moon, wind, water and fire), or man-made things (like houses, boats and cars), or even abstract forms (like numbers, or the triangle, the square, and the circle). In fact the whole cosmos is a potential symbol.

(Jung 1978: 257)

The photograph album is a treasure-house of symbols. Within it we see many images of our self, a self which is signified by the photograph in a way that makes it available for our objective scrutiny.

Understanding personal symbols through photographs

We all have special, personal symbols, those that are most meaningful for us, and that occur most commonly in our dreams and paintings. Therapists themselves need to identify the photographic symbols that are most significant for them, to understand the depth of meaning associated with these symbols, and to experience their power to activate feelings and memories.

What do our photographs signify about ourselves and our lives? Which photographs would we choose to symbolise aspects of our experience?

Maggie has a photograph which is highly significant for her in a symbolic way. She took a hauntingly beautiful photograph of her children (Photograph 31) on a visit to the grave of her mother, who had died many years ago. It may be apparent that the picture describes much more than two children in a churchyard, but only Maggie herself can explain the exact nature of the personal symbols.

For her, the photograph was a poignant way of connecting her mother and her children, who, sadly, had never known each other. There is a symbolic contrast between the young lives, full of potential, and the finality of death. The picture symbolises an internal 'meeting' for Maggie, a linking of past and present, a way of signifying the circle of death and life:

See, I took the children to meet her. I think that they looked like angels in the picture. There is an aura, around their heads, a reflection. There are double images, shadows, in the picture. The sun shone down on us all. . . . It was a perfect day.

The images are symbolic of Maggie's wish to integrate old and new, life and death, and to move towards wholeness.

Developing symbolic thinking

In order to be able to use photographic symbolism and metaphor to benefit both self and patient, therapists need to develop the ability to think symbolically.

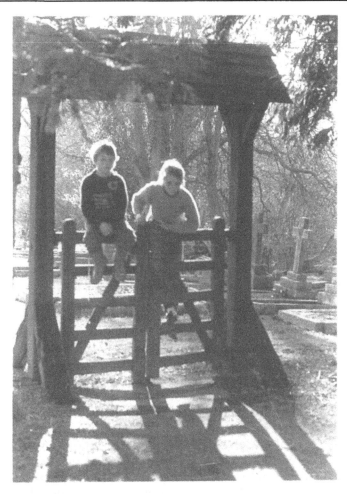

Photograph 31
© Maggie Wilson

This will necessitate an awareness that any image in a photograph may have deep and symbolic personal meaning; such an approach involves an openness to the gradual emergence of this meaning.

Dr Robert Hobson, after Jung, calls this the 'symbolical attitude':

At this point, my task . . . is not to explain but to attend; to remain in touch with, and to value, the experience as intimating what is as yet unknown. To be ready to receive what will emerge and lead forward. Following Jung, I have called this expectant waiting, a symbolical attitude.

(Hobson 1985: 35)

Symbols and metaphors in therapy

Symbolic images in therapy may expand into metaphors. These provide us with ways of describing an experience in terms of an image that is apparently unconnected, yet is inventively linked through the medium of the metaphor. In this way, there is often facilitated a new and creative understanding, a clarification.

The use of both metaphor and symbol in psychotherapy is very widespread and important; it is a potent communicational tool. The photograph, too, may be seen as metaphorical, and sometimes patients may present pictures that are overtly so; these are offered as a way of explaining, and managing, difficult issues.

Kate's use of a photographic metaphor will serve to illustrate how powerful is this medium in helping us all – patients and therapists alike – to learn more about our selves, past and present.

Kate, now in her thirties, showed me a greying, monochromatic photograph of her snow-covered garden, which she had taken at the age of 16. This was a very unhappy time in her life, and she felt lonely and unheard, constantly in tears.

On the day she took the picture, she had made a decision not to cry again; no one noticed her tears anyway. The mournfulness of the picture, she felt, represented the pain of the decision. Taking the picture had been an attempt to externalise inner feelings in a way that she found difficult verbally, for words had been largely unheard in her childhood, so she had learned to suppress them. Kate had been a lonely, desperate girl, who had spontaneously used the photographic process in an attempt to heal and comfort herself in a painful world.

She may have also used the picture to reflect her inner pain in a way that her family could not do, to give it an image outside herself, have it seen, if only through the eye of the camera. At least then it existed outside herself, even if there were no human being to confirm and reflect it.

Bringing this photograph into therapy, and using it as a metaphor for her pain, helped her remember and relive the traumatic feelings she had experienced as a child. She had great difficulty in showing her feelings in therapy, especially at the beginning, and the photograph was her way of offering to me some inkling of how difficult it had been for her.

Up to this point, it had been very hard for Kate to show me any of her inner self, or any of the considerable creativity that she was too afraid to reveal. The photograph told me – and perhaps reminded Kate, too – of the sensitivity and imaginative ability that lay behind a somewhat blank exterior in terms of feelings.

Somehow it made it easier than before for me to empathise with her and to be aware of what lay behind the rather off-putting defence. Previously, there had been little to relate to, for she had seemed so cut-off, so unemotional. She was presenting me with a visual metaphor of her depression and suffering, a grey picture of a snowy garden, that graphically represented the frozen inner garden of her soul. The photograph was a poignant statement about herself, framed within a metaphor. Through it, life was again breathed into the petrified feelings, for Kate cried as she re-experienced the depths of her adolescent turmoil. The photographic metaphor had provided a way into the unconscious.

Sameness and difference

The use of photographic symbolism can facilitate connectedness between two people; for there is universal as well as a personal aspect to many of these symbols. Understanding my own personal symbols is linked to understanding those from within another person's secret world. Familiar symbols emerge from the collective unconscious (Jung 1978); these are shared images with universal meanings, known to us all.

Photographs can, as we have seen, emphasise that there is a family of man and woman, as we note the resemblances and similarities within the albums of another person, who is a part of the same world as ourselves:

> Thus we will see people as constantly being born, changing and finally passing away. Everyone is subject to the cycle of birth and death, and because of this, everyone in the universe is as *One* being. Thus, seeing one person clearly and distinctly is the same as seeing every person in the world.
>
> (Chan Ajahn 1982: 30)

The person to be seen most clearly, for the therapist, needs to be the self; only then can she really see another and respond and reflect empathically.

However, as well as underlining the connectedness of all humanity, photographic symbolism may be seen as confirming the uniqueness of the individual. As therapists, we therefore need to be able also to differentiate between the symbols that are most meaningful for us, and those of the patient.

Photographs of a patient's family can sometimes make it easier for the therapist to separate the other's issues from her own, because she can see the very apparent differences before her in the pictures. Nevertheless, coincidences and resemblances may reactivate feelings and memories about past issues in the therapist's life; the symbols and metaphors in a patient's photographs may trigger the therapist's own personal ones.

Thus the therapist's vision may become obscured by her own projections onto the patient's images. Plaut speaks of the therapist's imagination sometimes creating imagery for the patient (Plaut 1966: 121). Just as there is a danger that the therapist may be carried away by her own verbal inventiveness and put words into the patient's mouth, so the therapist can put images into the patient's head that will, in fact, indicate more about herself.

Whilst it is never possible to have absolutely pure vision, it is important that the therapist clarifies her personal issues and delineates their boundaries, so that themes from her own symbolic world will not become confused with and superimposed upon the patient's.

How can the therapist ensure that her way of looking is relatively uncontaminated by personal material? Very often, one of the motivations for becoming a therapist will have been to learn more about the self, to aid the therapist's own self-discovery – and this is as it should be.

In order to differentiate between self and patient, however, the therapist needs to ensure that she herself has an adequate support system in terms of supervision and her own therapy. Through engaging in these, and becoming familiar with her photographic symbols and images, she will be able to empathise, but not over-identify, with the patient.

'PLAYING' WITH PHOTOGRAPHS TO INCREASE SELF-KNOWLEDGE

Photographs help us know more about ourselves and the world. Through playing with these images, and thinking openly and creatively, we may devise ways of using them to enhance our self-awareness. The ideas and exercises here are merely a way of stimulating the readers of this book to think about the area for themselves; readers will no doubt devise more ways of working personally with photographs as they learn to become more creative with their pictures.

The symbolic function of the photograph enables a firm distance to be maintained from the disturbing realities of our selves and our lives. The self is objectified by the photograph as signifier; its inanimate security may make it less risky for us to experiment with our self-image. In order to objectify the self-image even further, for purposes of detachment and clarity, it is often helpful to look at the reflected photograph in a mirror (Wessels 1985: 96).

Different angles on the self

In Chapter 2, I discussed the need for flexibility of thought and attitude, in order to discover the many paradoxes within the photograph. Maybe you will now want to endeavour to find the hidden opposites and contradictions inside yourself. Having almost reached the end of this book, you may now feel ready to begin to experiment with aspects of your own self-image through photographs.

Perhaps you can start, in fantasy, to turn yourself inside out, upside down, see yourself in reverse and from above, having practised the art of flexible thinking. Photographs are an excellent help in this; for nowhere else, except in moving pictures, can we see ourselves from behind, in profile, from above, or upside down. Unlike the reflection we see in a mirror, our image in a photograph is not laterally inverted, so we really do see ourselves as others see us; but we also do not, because, paradoxically, it is 'just' a photograph of ourselves that we see.

In gaining greater insight into the self, whether in therapy or in our lives in general, it is important to see ourselves from many different angles. Photographs can help us to see the whole picture of ourselves on an emotional level, as well as on a physical one.

Split self pictures

Yoka, photographer and counsellor, worked with me on some interesting photographic exercises, in order to find out more about the different sides of herself. She had a friend take some close-up photographs of her face, showing her with many different poses and with a variety of facial expressions, from all angles. She then pasted some of the pictures on a board, to show a collection of moods and expressions. Others, she cut up in various ways, putting, for example, a group of eyes or mouths together, noting the differences, looking at the shapes, and the 'statement' made by each photograph. She was surprised to discover the many faces and characters within her self.

Most interestingly, she cut a full-face photograph in half, put aside one half, then reversed the other and photographed this. She then put the real half and the reversed half together and made a total 'right side' picture of her face and a total 'left side' picture. If this is difficult to imagine, look at the results, in Photographs 32 and 33. See how the two halves of the face differ, so that Yoka can discover something of the hidden, partial selves within her that constitute her total self.

Yoka's feelings about and projections onto the split side photographs are most revealing in terms of her self-image. Let us see what she has to say:

I think the right side (Photograph 32) is my ugly side, fleshy and big – but it is also happy. I would have expected the left side (Photograph 33) to be happy, but it is not. It is prettier and smoother, though. That shows me that real happiness and beauty is from the inside, not dependent on superficialities. I think the right side is more at ease, it does not have to try to be anything other than it is. It has completely come to terms with being ugly; this is the part of me that is happy being myself. The left side is more serious, discontented and expresses my feelings of striving for things I don't get.

It is paradoxical that the right side looks more like my mother, and the narrow, left side is more my father. Yet my father is the happier of the two!

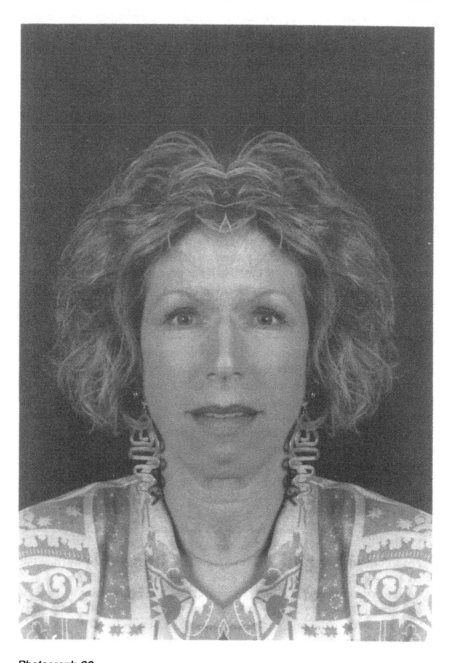

Photograph 32

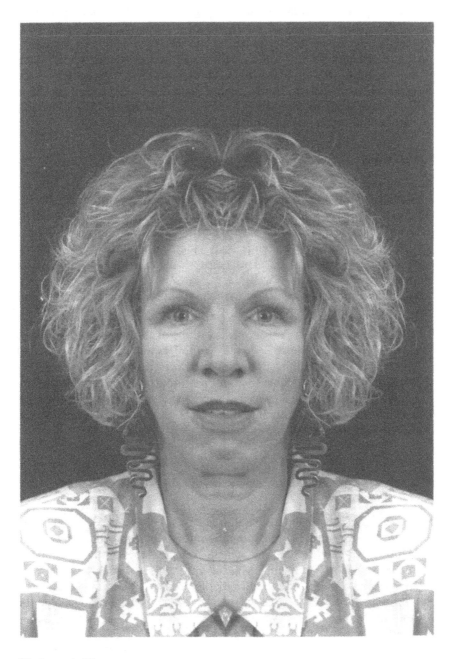

Photograph 33

I like my 'selves' more than I thought I would. I can't get over the different sizes of nose. In the right side picture, my nose is big. That is what I used to see when I looked at myself, especially as a teenager. Now I've changed sides! I see only the small, left side nose when I look at a photograph. It's all a matter of perception. The right side is more extravert. I like it better. I think my left side is a bit depressed. Perhaps I don't really want to face those feelings . . . maybe this is saying that I've looked on the bright side for too long, denied the negatives.

Self-portraits

As mentioned in Chapter 3, the making of self-portraits with the camera provides an extra dimension and allows people to contrast present self with child self. Exploring one's photographic self-portrait as a therapist or patient is a powerful and vivid way of clarifying feelings about self-image.

Additionally, one may examine body language, and the pose, noticing how it alters over the years. This helps to understand more about the internal world.

Ziller encourages people to use the camera to explore self and environment:

> The self-concept derives from observations of the self by the self. The study of self-concept is the search for understanding of ourselves and others. But understanding of the self requires a mode of communication about our self-observations that will not obfuscate the response to the query: 'Who am I?' It is proposed here that iconic communication with a camera will produce images of the self that avoid some of the shortcomings of verbal self-reports.
>
> (Ziller 1990: 28)

'Changing the portrait': some active therapeutic work with family photographs

Maggie wanted to find out more about herself and her inner world through photographs, to capture some authentic interactions on camera by having herself photographed 'behind the scenes'. Taking the risk of being captured on film in her 'worst' moments, Maggie was influenced in this by the work of Jo Spence, who used the camera to explore herself and the world in an insightful and real way. Jo Spence asks: 'How can we begin to change the portrait, to change ideas of what should and should not go into our family albums?' (Spence 1986: 94).

Maggie had been troubled by some recent anger towards her daughter, Alice, and she had them both act out an angry scenario for the camera.

Through such photographs, and using me as her colleague/helper, she was able to make a crucial link. She saw that the anger towards her daughter was connected to unresolved feelings about her own mother and her mother's death, which occurred when Maggie was 22. The photographs triggered memories of her own childhood relationship with mother, when Maggie had felt her anger was repressed and that many of her needs were unmet.

Maggie now came to understand that Alice was angry with her for moving the family to England, away from all that was dear and familiar to her in Australia. This was a kind of loss, and mirrored the feelings that Maggie had towards *her* mother for not meeting her needs and for dying young:

> We're both experiencing a similar type of anger, aren't we . . . anger about loss . . . looking at this photo helps me see the link. My first arguments with my mother were when I was the age Alice is now. . . . I think I was really also angry with Mother for keeping such control of her anger. She never stood up for herself. Am I angry with Mother for being so passive? Am I using Alice as an outlet for that pent-up anger? My mother let me carry all her angry feelings – I wanted to push her away.

She then realised, as she looked at the picture reconstruction of herself shaking Alice, that she was wanting to push her, too (Photograph 34). Alice is, in fact smiling, but Maggie remembers feeling real anger.

It seemed difficult, though, for Maggie to get in touch with her own childhood anger and to hear it, just as it was not heard at the time. In fact, she was now punishing a child, Alice, for being angry.

There was thus a most confusing and confused jumble of images and feelings that emerged in relation to herself, her inner child, her daughter and her mother. They were bound together with grief and anger, and the feelings and projections were hard to separate and see clearly.

'Such stuff as dreams are made on . . .'

The photographs that Maggie had reconstructed were visual projections of her internal self, like remnants of stilled dreams. Symbolically, she had used herself and Alice as actors on the stage of her inner world. I wondered if the inner juxtaposition and confusion could somehow be expressed externally by manipulating the photographs.

Could she, perhaps, superimpose various internal figures (her mother, herself as a child) onto the people in this picture, to bring the fantasies alive, to create the stuff of dreams? Could she use her energy to transform the inner view of the past into something creative, rather than destructive? This kind of exercise is very akin to Gestalt dreamwork, where dreamers are urged to work on, and have power over, their dreams, thus changing the course of their waking life.

The results of Maggie's subsequent photographic creativity led to

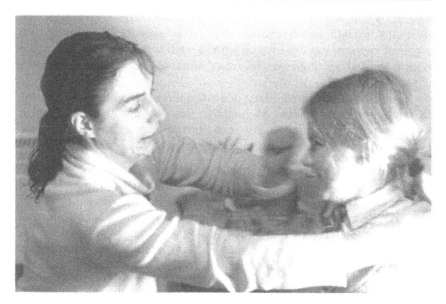

Photograph 34
© Maggie Wilson

increased clarity and understanding for Maggie. Whilst doing these exercises, she had focused on untangling past and present feelings and, in doing so, had learned to differentiate between Alice and herself.

In Photograph 35 there is an empty space where Alice had been. Maggie saw this space as having potential, because she could project anyone in the family into it. In fact, there is in the original print still a ghost, a trace of Alice left in the picture. This was a mistake, but we wondered what it represented: could this be the ghost of Maggie's own inner child, or perhaps the spectre of her anger? She wondered if she had unconsciously wanted a ghost there.

Subsequently, she experimented with that space, for it had considerable potential in terms of playing and fantasy. She imagined several people in it, projecting onto the picture other members of her family whom she might want to shake in the way she had shaken Alice. Then she tried to fill the space with a shadowy, superimposed picture of herself at about 9, a similar age to Alice. Maggie was really able to feel, through doing this, how distressing it would be to have a big aggresssive adult shake her in that way. She reflected that the photographs had helped her see just how much anger she had been carrying for and towards her mother, and that she was acting this out with her own daughter.

Maggie also saw how her adult self became angry with the inner child self, already overburdened with carrying the weight of her own and her

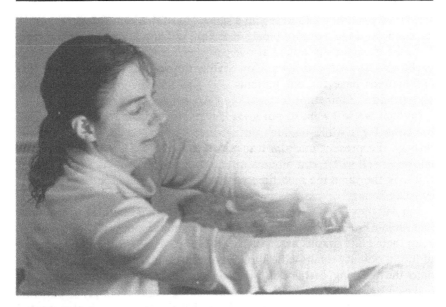

Photograph 35
© Maggie Wilson

mother's repressed anger. She learned to be more accepting of this inner child, to nurture her rather than punish her, to allow her to express grief and anger.

Maggie found that her anger had reduced, and had 'perhaps been transformed'. She now realised that, as a child, she had been locked into the caring role with her mother, so that her own needs were repressed. Maggie's anger lessened as she was able to connect with the inner needy child: 'I discovered the unheard demanding child within me, which seemed compelled to press others into my service.' Maggie's work with photographs revealed to her just how much she had repeated inherited patterns; through the understanding thus promoted, she was able to find another way of being.

Journey's end: contemplating impermanence

The purpose of this chapter has been to encourage a focus on the self-image through photographs, and to re-view our own albums in the light of new ideas, new challenges.

As we have done so, we have inevitably come face to face with our own history. Dead moments may suddenly have pulsed into life, jolting us into recollections of the self that we once were. It may be difficult, having begun such a journey, to orient ourselves in the present, to close these albums of yesterday and to regain a sense of self in time. The photographs have removed the memory blocks that kept us fixed in the present so that, from the moment we looked at our early pictures, we were sent tumbling backwards through our lives. How vividly do we thus feel the power that photographs have for our patients . . . how much more clearly can we understand the immense force of their experiences.

Perhaps we will want to put away our photographs now, to firmly close the book for a while on such disturbance. As we do so, ready to move through the present into the future, we can surely be confident that the images of self within our albums will be statically preserved, and that they will look the same the next time we come to view them, perhaps months, or years hence.

But will they? Can we really be certain that there is anything in existence that remains immutable, held in a state of infinite sameness? Often, people keep their photographs as a kind of insurance against the impermanence of life, a defence against the threat of change and loss, a way of holding onto the pleasing certainties that have been. And yet the photograph makes no promises that we will remain as we were. It simply documents *how* we were. In retrospect, we will see that the photograph represented a moment in transit.

The closed mind, resistant to new ways of being, afraid of uncertainty, will see only the superficially fixed photographic images. As therapists, we need to be open to change, to move forward through processes of knowledge and self-awareness. Then, transformations will be seen to occur within our static collections of images.

Photographs, which reflect our ever-changing lives, are inevitably a part of them; as such, they are not exempt from life's impermanence. They, too, change. The meanings of these apparently secure images are fixed only in our inner experience of them.

Conclusion

I have endeavoured in this book to reveal some of the tantalising, puzzling and fascinating qualities of the photograph. Enigmatic, sometimes enticingly cryptic, photographs inspire us to poetry and prose, to artistic and academic study, philosophical debate and psychological enquiry. We have seen above all how they can be a stimulus to memory and emotion; charade-like glimpses of reality, crystallised for posterity, they have presented us here with life in all its richness and intricacy.

I have illustrated how photographs may be a valuable adjunct to many therapeutic processes and can thus be used to powerful effect. I have proposed that they may also have much to teach us in our lives generally, if we can adopt a more creative manner of looking at them. They may then be used to expand rather than restrict the mind's potential.

I trust that I have communicated something of the importance of the potential role of photographs in therapy of all kinds. Those who have seen photographs as merely superficial images may have been encouraged to think again. I hope that therapists will be more inclined to perceive photographs as a potentially useful tool in therapy and to widen their way of seeing.

I have emphasised in this book the power of the image, and also the fact that the capacity to use the image, for good or for evil, lies within us. If I have had one aim above all others, it has been to stimulate people to realise that they can choose to use the photographic image therapeutically.

At the very end of the process of psychotherapy, the intention is that the patient will have internalised a good enough image of the therapist to enable him or her to move forward through life with strength and hope. *My* hope, at the very end of this book, is that you, the reader, will have internalised some of its images and reflections, with a view to using them for healing, for insight and for understanding.

Notes

PREFACE

1 The term 'photo-therapy' may be defined thus: 'the use of photography or photographic materials, under the guidance of a trained therapist, to reduce or relieve painful psychological symptoms and to facilitate psychological growth and therapeutic change' (Stewart 1979: 42).

1 PHOTOGRAPHS IN EVERYDAY LIFE

1 Extract from the 'Kodacolor Gold' Survey, April 1990, prepared by Audience Selection, London for Kodak Limited.
2 This is a quotation from an essay written by Lewis Hine in 1909 entitled 'Social Photography: How the Camera May Help in the Social Uplift'. It was delivered at a session of an annual meeting of the National Conference of Charities and Correction.
   This information is from an essay by A. Trachtenberg (1977: 133) in *America & Lewis Hine*. In this book the Foreword is by Walter Rosenblum and biographical notes by Naomi Rosenblum.

2 PARADOXES AND THE PHOTOGRAPH

1 Shorter Oxford English Dictionary.
2 'Ceci n'est pas une pipe', by René Magritte. In the collection of William Copley, New York.

4 A CLINICAL EXAMPLE

1 Morning suit in Photograph 11 courtesy of Silhouette Dress Service, Ltd., Taylor and Cross, Altrincham, Cheshire.

6 EXPLORING IMAGES OF INTERACTION

1 Quoted from a Channel 4 programme, *Opening up the Family Album*, August 1988. Produced by John Ellis at Large Door Ltd. Series concept: Jo Spence. Director: Nina Kellgren.

7 WHO CAN BENEFIT?

1 Freud, too, must have understood the therapeutic power of the photograph after termination. Kardiner, who had just completed analysis with Freud relates:

My analysis terminated on the first of April 1922. I felt uneasy, reluctant to leave, and, in a way, resentful about it. I asked Freud for an autographed photograph, which he gave me. On it he wrote in German, 'To Dr. A. Kardiner – as a friendly remembrance of his sojourn in Vienna – Freud.'

(Kardiner 1977: 67–8)

2 I am grateful for some of this information to Dr Colin Murray-Parkes.

3 There are therapeutic facilities for Holocaust survivors in the London area. Contact Judith Hassan at Shalvata (081–203–9033) for more information.

4 Written by Margaret Bourke-White, in a letter to *Life* magazine, May 1945.

5 Whilst I am very well aware that both men and women suffer sexual abuse in childhood, I have referred to the abuse survivor as 'she'. This is for clarity only, and in no way implies that there are not male survivors.

6 The concept of the inner child originated in the work of Alice Miller (1987). Some of the ways of working with the inner child were inspired by Parks (1990).

Bibliography

Akeret, R.V. (1973) *Photoanalysis*, New York, Peter H. Wyden.

Ammerman, M.S. and Fryrear, J.L. (1975) 'Photographic enhancement of children's self-esteem', *Psychology in the Schools* 12 (3), 319–25.

Arguile, R. (1990) '"I show you": children in art therapy', in C. Case and T. Dalley (eds) *Working with Children in Art Therapy*, London, Tavistock/Routledge.

Barthes, R. (1988) [1980] *Camera Lucida*, London, Fontana.

Benjamin, W. (1972) [1931] 'A short history of photography', *Screen* 13 (1), 5–26.

Berner, J. (1975) *The Photographic Experience*, New York, Anchor Books.

Blue, L. (1985) [1979] *A Backdoor to Heaven*, London, Fount.

Bonime, W. (1962) *The Clinical Use of Dreams*, New York, Basic Books.

Bourdieu, P. (1990) *Photography, A Middle-Brow Art*, translated by Shaun Whiteside, Cambridge, Polity Press.

Brandon, D. (1976) *Zen in the Art of Helping*, London, Routledge & Kegan Paul.

Byng-Hall, J. (1979) 'Re-editing family mythology during family therapy', *Journal of Family Therapy* 1, 103–16.

Casement, P. (1985) *On Learning from the Patient*, London, Tavistock.

Champlin, T.S. (1988) *Reflexive Paradoxes*, London, Routledge.

Chan Ajahn, The Venerable (1982) *Budhinyana*, Thailand, Funny Press.

Doyle, M. (1976) *Stonedancer*, Australia, University of Auckland Bindery.

Entin, A.D. (1982) 'Family icons: photographs in family psychotherapy', in L.E. Abt and I.R. Stuart (eds) *The Newer Therapies. A Sourcebook*, New York, Van Nostrand Reinhold.

Ferreira, A.J. (1963) 'Family myth and homeostasis', *Archives of General Psychiatry* 9, 457–63.

Fraser, S. (1989) [1987] *My Father's House*, London, Virago.

Friday, N. (1983) [1977] *My Mother, My Self*, London, Fontana.

Fryrear, J.L. and Corbit, I.E. (1989) 'Visual transitions – metaphor for change', in H. Wadeson, J. Durkin and D. Perach (eds) *Advances in Art Therapy*, New York, Wiley.

Fryrear, J.L., Neull, L.R. and White, P. (1977) 'Enhancement of male juvenile delinquents' self-concepts through photographed social interactions', *Journal of Clinical Psychology* 33 (3), 833–8.

Gottheil, E., Backup, C.E. and Cornelison, F.S. (1969) 'Denial and self-image confrontation in a case of anorexia nervosa', *Journal of Nervous and Mental Disease* 148 (3), 238–50.

Grass, G. (1962) [1959] *The Tin Drum*, London, Secker & Warburg.

Hafner, R.J. (1986) *Marriage and Mental Illness*, New York, Guilford Press.

Hall, L. and Lloyd, S. (1989) *Surviving Child Sexual Abuse*, London, Falmer Press.
Hobson, R.F. (1985) *Forms of Feeling*, London, Tavistock Publications.
Hogan, P.T. (1981) 'Phototherapy in the educational setting', *The Arts in Psychotherapy* 8, 193–9.
Holmes, J. (1985) 'The language of psychotherapy: metaphor, ambiguity, wholeness', *British Journal of Psychotherapy* 1 (4), 240–54.
Jennings, S. (1973) *Remedial Drama*, London, Pitman.
Jung, C.G. (1977) [1925] 'The development of the personality', *Collected Works* 17, London, Routledge & Kegan Paul.
—— (1978) [1964] *Man and His Symbols*, London, Picador.
Kardiner, A. (1977) *My Analysis with Freud*, New York, Norton.
Kohut, H. (1979) 'The two analyses of Mr Z.', *International Journal of Psycho-Analysis* 60 (3), 3–27.
Kopp, S. (1980) [1972] *If You Meet Buddha on the Road, Kill Him!* London, Sheldon Press.
Krauss, D.A. (1980) 'A summary of characteristics of photographs which make them useful in counseling and therapy', *Camera Lucida* 1 (2), 7–11.
Krell, R. (1990) 'Holocaust survivors: a clinical perspective', *Psychiatric Journal University of Ottawa* 15 (1), 18–21.
Lichfield, P. (1981) *Lichfield on Photography*, London, Collins.
Love, P. (1990) *The Emotional Incest Syndrome*, New York, Bantam.
Masayesva, V. and Younger, E. (1984) [1983] *Hopi Photographers, Hopi Images*, Tucson, University of Arizona Press.
McKinney, J.P. (1979) 'Photo counseling', *Children Today* 8, 29.
McRea, C. (1983) 'Impact on body-image', in P.W. Dowrick and S.J. Biggs (eds) *Using Video*, New York, Wiley.
Milgram, S. (1977) *The Individual in a Social World*, Massachusetts, Addison-Wesley.
Miller, A. (1987) [1980] *For Your Own Good – The Roots of Violence in Child-rearing*, London, Virago.
Milner, M. (1977) [1950] *On Not Being Able to Paint*, London, Heinemann.
Morris, D. (1986) *The Pocket Guide to Manwatching*, London, Triad Grafton Books.
Nathan, L. (1982) *Holding Patterns*, Pittsburgh, University of Pittsburgh Press.
Newlin, M. (1973) *Day of Sirens*, Manchester, Carcanet; also published in *Collected Poems 1963–1985*, Michigan, Ardis (1986).
Ortony, A. (1975) 'Why metaphors are necessary and not just nice', *Educational Theory* 25, 45–53.
Parks, P. (1990) *Rescuing the Inner Child*, London, Souvenir Press.
Perls, F., Hefferline, R.F. and Goodman, P. (1951) *Gestalt Therapy: Excitement and Growth in the Human Personality*, New York, Dell.
Plaut, A. (1966) 'Reflections About Not Being Able to Imagine', *Journal of Analytical Psychology* 11 (2), 113–33.
Pollock, G.H. (1981) 'Reminiscences and insight', *The Psychoanalytic Study of the Child* 36, 279–87.
Proust, M. (1981) [1954] *Remembrance of Things Past*, vol. 1, *Swann's Way*, London, Chatto & Windus.
Radford, E. and Radford, M.A. (1961) *Encyclopaedia of Superstitions*. C. Hole (ed.), London, Hutchinson.
Reps, P. (ed.) (1989) [1957] *Zen Flesh, Zen Bones*, Rutland, VT, Charles E. Tuttle.
Rodger, G. (1987) *Magnum Opus*, London, Dirk Nishen Publishing.
Rosten, L. (1977) [1972] *Treasury of Jewish Quotations*, New York, Bantam.

Sartre, J.P. (1957) [1943] *Being and Nothingness*, London, Methuen.

Searles, H. (1960) *The Non-Human Environment*, Monograph series on Schizophrenia 5, New York, International University Press.

Sontag, S. (1987) [1977] *On Photography*, Penguin, London.

Spalding, H.D. (1969) *Encyclopedia of Jewish Humor*, New York, Jonathan David.

Spence, J. (1986) *Putting Myself in the Picture*, London, Camden Press.

Stewart, D. (1979) 'Photo-therapy: theory and practice', *Art Psychotherapy* 6, 41–6.

Thomas, R.S. (1978) 'Album', in *Frequencies*, London, Macmillan University Press.

Trachtenberg, A. (1977) *America & Lewis Hine*, New York, Aperture.

—— (ed.) (1980) *Classic Essays on Photography*, New Haven, CT, Leete's Island Books.

Vishniac, R. (1983) *A Vanished World*, New York, Farrar, Straus & Giroux.

Volkan, V.D., Cilluffo, A.F. and Sarvay, T.L. Jr (1976) 'Re-grief therapy and the function of the linking object as a key to stimulate emotionality', in P. Olsen (ed.) *Emotional Flooding*, vol. 1 of *New Directions in Psychotherapy*, New York, Human Sciences Press.

Wadeson, H., Durkin, J. and Perach, D. (eds) (1989) *Advances in Art Therapy*, New York, Wiley.

Watzlawick, P., Weakland, J. and Fisch, R. (1974) *Change*, New York, W. Norton.

Weiser, J. (1988) '"See what I mean?" Photography as nonverbal communication in cross-cultural psychology', in F. Poyatos (ed.) *Cross-Cultural Perspectives in Nonverbal Communication*, Toronto, Hogrefe.

—— (1990) 'The Secret Lives of Snapshots', *Canadian Living*, November, 115–21.

Wessels, D.T. (1985) 'Using family photographs in the treatment of eating disorders', *Psychotherapy in Private Practice*, 3 (4), 95–105.

Wilson, M. (1991) 'The photograph as signifier and its use in therapy', unpublished dissertation, Dip. in Art Therapy, Goldsmiths' College, London.

Winnicott, D.W. (1958) [1935] 'The manic defence', in *Collected Papers: Through Paediatrics to Psychoanalysis*, London, Tavistock Publications.

—— (1991) *Human Nature*, London, Free Association Books.

Wordsworth, W. (1968) [1805] 'The tables turned', in D. Roper (ed.) *Wordsworth and Coleridge: Lyrical Ballads*, London, Collins.

Zilbach, J.J. (1986) *Young Children in Family Therapy*, New York, Brunner/Mazel.

Ziller, R.C. (1990) *Photographing the Self*, California, Sage Publications.

Ziller, R.C. and Smith, R.A. (1977) 'A phenomenological utilization of photographs', *Journal of Phenomenological Psychology* 7 (2), 172–82.

Further reading

Beloff, H. (1985) *Camera Culture*, New York, Basil Blackwell.

Berger, J. (1980) *About Looking*, London, Writers and Readers Publishing Cooperative.

Butler, R.N. (1963) 'The life review: an interpretation of reminiscence in the aged', *Psychiatry* 26, 65–76.

Combs, J.M. and Ziller, R.C. (1977) 'Photographic self-concept of counsellees', *Journal of Counselling Psychology* 24 (5), 452–5.

Entin, A.S. (1981) 'The use of photographs and family albums in family therapy', in Alan Gurman (ed.) *Questions and Answers in the Practice of Family Therapy*, New York, Brunner/Mazel.

Evans, H. (1990) *Headline Photography*, London, Treasure Press.

Hattersley, R. (1971) *Discover Your Self through Photography*, New York, Association Press.

Kaslow, F.W. and Friedman, J. (1977) 'Utilization of family photos and movies in family therapy', *Journal of Marriage and Family Counselling* 3, 19–25.

Martin, R. and Spence, J. (1988) 'Photo-therapy: psychic realism as healing art?' *Ten-8* 30, 3–17.

Milton, S. (1984) 'The camera as weapon: documentary photography and the holocaust', *Simon Wiesenthal Centre Annual* 1, 45–63.

Spence, J. and Holland, P. (eds) (1991) *Family Snaps: The Meanings of Domestic Photography*, London, Virago.

Titus, S.L. (1976) 'Family photographs and transition to parenthood', *Journal of Marriage and the Family* 38 (3), 525–30.

Weiser, J. (1990) 'More than meets the eye: using ordinary snapshots as tools for therapy', in Toni Laidlaw, Cheryl Malmo and associates (eds) *Healing Voices: Feminist Approaches to Therapy with Women*, San Francisco, Jossey Bass.

Williamson, J. (1977) 'Family, education and photography', *Ten-8* 14, 19–22.

Wolf, R. (1976) 'The polaroid technique: spontaneous dialogues from the unconscious', *Art Psychotherapy* 3, 197–214.

Ziller, R.C. and Lewis, D. (1981) 'Orientations: self, social and environmental percepts through auto-photography', *Personality and Social Psychology Bulletin* 7 (2), 338–43.

Name index

Abells, H. 15
Akeret, R.V. 68
Ammerman, M.S. 150
Arbus, D. 37
Arguile, R. 152–3

Backup, C.E. 155
Barthes, R. 14–15, 17, 25
Benjamin, W. 122
Berner, J. 8–9
Blue, L. 38
Bonime, W. 101
Bourdieu, P. 7–8
Bourke-White, M. 162
Brandon, D. 24, 38
Byng-Hall, J. 134

Casement, P. 62
Champlin, T.S. 29
Chan Ajahn, The Venerable 193
Cooper, T. 26
Corbit, I.E. 144, 148, 153
Cornelison, F.S. 155

Daguerre, L. 2
Dodd, K. 33
Doyle, M. 174

Entin, A.D. 144
Epictetus 48

Ferreira, A.J. 133–4
Fox, C. 181–2
Franz, K. 20
Fraser, S. 37–8
Freud, S. 204–5
Friday, N. 188
Fryrear, J.L. 150
Fuller, R. Buckminster 8

Gatenby, D. 33
Gottheil, E. 155
Grass, G. 105

Hafner, R.J. 178
Hall, L. 164, 165, 168
Hine, L. 204
Hobson, R.F. 50, 191
Hogan, P.T. 150
Holmes, J. 43

Ibn Gabirol 63
Ibn Zabara 35

Jennings, S. 154
Jung, C.G. 27–8, 137–8, 189–90, 191, 193

Kardiner, A. 204–5
Kaye, G. 20
Kohut, H. 114–15
Kopp, S. 103
Krauss, D.A. 53
Krell, R. 162

Lichfield, P. 108
Lloyd, S. 164, 165, 168
Love, P. 136

McKinney, J.P. 150
McRea, C. 155
Magritte, R. 29
Masayesva, V. 19
Milgram, S. 17, 132, 186
Miller, A. 3, 205
Milligan, L. 155
Milner, M. 44
Morris, D. 11–12

Nathan, L. 51
Newlin, M. 1

Ortony, A. 12

Parks, P. 205
Perls, F. 46
Plaut, A. 69, 193
Pollock, G.H. 146
Proust, M. 55

Radford, E. 16
Radford, M.A. 16
Reps, P. 49
Rodger, G. 36–7
Rosten, L. 35, 63
Rudkin, A. 33

Sartre, J.P. 182
Searles, H. 96
Smith, R.A. 152
Sontag, S. 16–17, 37, 82, 146

Spalding, H.D. 6
Spence, J. 133, 198
Stewart, D. 204

Thomas, R.S. 23
Trachtenberg, A. 3

Vishniac, R. 12
Volkan, V.D. 159

Wadeson, H. 144, 149
Watzlawick, P. 48
Weiser, J. 119, 156
Wessels, D.T. 154, 194
Wilson, M. 111–12, 178–80, 190–1,
   198–201
Winnicott, D.W. 3, 67–8, 116
Wordsworth, W. 60

Younger, E. 19

Zilbach, J.J. 144
Ziller, R.C. 52, 152, 198

Subject index

abuse, sexual *see* sexual abuse
acceptable/unacceptable selves 39, 40
adolescents, photo-therapy with 149
adoption process, use of photographs in 150–1
album, family: construction 53; family myth 132–5; function 105–6; omissions 111–13; in therapy 106–13
amnesia, treatment of 148
anger, expression of 167–8
anorexia nervosa 154, 155–6
art therapy 152–3

beauty of photographs 37
behaviour patterns *see* patterns
Belsen photographs 36–7, 161
bereavement 156–9
birth order 118–19
Buchenwald photographs 162

catharsis 100–1
child: inner 164–5; parental 135–6
children: in care 150–1; on display 6; holding 114–16; response to photographs 3–4; use of photographs in therapy 148–51
collective unconscious 27–8
communication 9–13; from past 113
conformity 180–5
control 4–5, 28
counter-transference 60, 70, 96–7

Daily Mirror 162
death and life 35
dementia 147–8

difference: meaningful 136–8; sameness and 193–4
display 6
double thinking 47
dynamics, family 131–45

eating disorders 154–6
eternity 15–16, 33

familiar and strange 30
family: abusing 163; dynamics and interaction 131–45; group 41; identification 27; myth 132–5; resemblances 187–8; roles and structures 135–6; therapy 143–5; *see also* album
fantasy and reality 26
Fox Ward, Sutton Hospital 147–8
fragmentation 33–5
freeze-frame images 129–31

handicap, physical 151–2
health, patterns of 114
Hillsborough disaster 13, 21, 162–3
holding 114–16
Holocaust photographs 14–16, 20, 36–7, 160–2; *see also* Warsaw Ghetto
holograms 80–1
Hopi Indians 19
house, image of 177

image(s): changing 188–9; cultural 178–80; freeze-frame 129–31; ideal 37; messages behind 113–21; paradoxical 39; of parents 188–9; power of 99–100; symbols 27
impermanence 32–3, 201–2
individuation 188–9

insight, search for 98–9
interaction, family 131–45
interventions, sensitive 62–3

learning 117; difficulties 151–2
lies, photographic 17–18
life and death 35
listening 116–17
'look, the' 120–1
looking, therapeutic 77–81
loss and bereavement 156–9

magic 16–17, 35–6
marital: interaction 123–31; therapy
    119–20, 129–31
masking behaviour 39–41
meaning 27; search for 58, 98–9
memories 37–8, 54–6
metaphors 192–3
mistakes, photographic 6–9

Nazi photography 14, 20, 160
newspaper photography 20–1, 162

paradoxes: photographic 24–38, 46–9;
    in therapy 38–46
partner, selection of 127–8
past messages 113, 121
patient: -leads 70–2; relationship with
    therapist 57–8
patterns of behaviour 121; repeated
    139–43
permanence and transience 32–3,
    201–2
photograph(s): absence 165–6; active
    use 169–72, 198–201; appeal 2–4; art
    therapy 152–3; bringing to therapy
    65–9; as communication 9–13; 'good'
    186; importance 2–4; as 'linking
    object' 159; as magic 16–17; patients
    making 52–3; playing with 194–202;
    as projectives 53; psychodrama
    153–4; psychological significance 2–9;
    reading 107–8, 113; reality and 17–18;
    revealing 166–7; selection by patients
    72–5; series of 108–9; showing
    process 75–7; therapeutic looking
    77–81; time and 13–16; use with
    children and adolescents 148–51; use
    in family therapy 143–5; use in
    psychoanalytic psychotherapy 54–81;
    use in therapy with survivors of
    traumatic experiences 159–72; use in
    treatment of eating disorders 154–6;
    see also album
'photographic look' 25
photo-therapy: approaches to
    51–4; assessment for 69–72
play 101–2; facilitating 63–4
pose: for camera 185–6; paradox in
    41–3
power 28–9
Press Council 20, 21
psychodrama 153–4
public and personal 27–8

reaction formation 39
reality 17–18, 26, 47
rebellion 4–5
reconstruction 33–5
re-editing 47–9
reflexive paradox 29–30
reframing 47–9
reminiscence therapy 146–8
resistance 97–8

sameness and difference 193–4
scapegoating 138
self: acceptable/unacceptable 39, 40;
    -acceptance 180–5; -image 150,
    155–6, 175–6, 194–8; incomplete 39;
    -knowledge 194–202; photographs
    and 174–202; portraits 198;
    reorientation 168–9
separation and individuation 188–9
sex-role stereotyping 177–8
sexual: abuse 163–72; problems 129
sibling relationships 118–19
socialisation 119–20
split self pictures 195–8
splitting 128–9
story telling 31–2
Sun 2, 20
Sunday Sport 20–1
Sutton Hospital, Surrey 147–8
symbolic thinking 190–1
symbols 27–8, 189–94

termination issues 102–4
therapist: own reflections 173;
    relationship with patient 57–8; role
    59–65; search for self 185–6
time 13–16; paradoxes 32–3

timing, being aware of 64–5
transference 44–5, 76–7, 96–7
traumatic experiences 159–72
triangular relationships 138–9
truth 17–18

unconscious, the 54–6; optical 122

Vietnam War 28

Warsaw Ghetto 12, 34; *see also*
    Holocaust photographs
working through 58–9
wounding and healing 36
wounding image 18–22

Milton Keynes UK
Ingram Content Group UK Ltd.
UKHW040100071024
449327UK00019B/693